DR. HOLISTIC TREATMENTS FOR ALL CONDITIONS

Naturally Relieve Diabetes, High Blood Pressure, Digestive Issues, Liver Detox, Kidney Conditions, Herpes, Lupus and More

4 Recipes for Healing Diabetes 44
   5. Cinnamon and Clove Tea 44
   6. Fenugreek Seed Smoothie 46
   7. Bitter Melon Stir-Fry 48
   8. Coriander and Ginger Soup 50

OVERCOMING LUPUS 52
What is Lupus and Its Symptoms 53
Dr. Sebi's Approach to Treating Lupus 54
Recommended Diet and Herbs 55
4 Recipes for Healing Lupus 57
   9. Lupus Anti-Inflammatory Smoothie 57
   10. Elderberry and Chamomile Soothing Gel 59
   11. Omega-3 Rich Vegetable Stew 61
   12. Ginger and Fennel Tea 63

LOWERING HIGH BLOOD PRESSURE 65
Causes and Symptoms of High Blood Pressure 66
Dietary and Lifestyle Recommendations 67
Natural Herbs and Remedies 69
4 Recipes to Reduce High Blood Pressure 71
   13. Dandelion Greens and Thyme Infusion 71
   14. Hibiscus and Lemon Tea 73
   15. Beetroot and Ginger Juice 75
   16. Celery and Cucumber Smoothie 77

COMBATING CANCER WITH NATURAL METHODS 79
Understanding Cancer from a Holistic Perspective 80
Dr. Sebi's Cancer Treatment Protocols 81
Detoxifying the Body to Prevent Cancer 83
Nutritional Recommendations for Cancer Patients 84
BONUS 87
4 Recipes for Healing Cancer 88
   17. Anti-Cancer Green Juice 88
   18. Kale and Sage Stir-Fry 90
   19. Mushroom and Nopales Soup 92
   20. Carrot and Ginger Smoothie 94

MANAGING INFLAMMATORY CONDITIONS 96
Understanding Inflammation and Its Causes 98
Anti-Inflammatory Foods and Herbs 100
Dr. Sebi's Recommendations for Inflammation 101

ADDRESSING KIDNEY DISEASES 103
Overview of Kidney Function and Diseases 104
Dr. Sebi's Approach to Healing the Kidneys 105
Herbs and Diet for Kidney Health 107
4 Recipes for Healing Kidney Diseases 109
21. Nettle and Dandelion Tea 109
22. Raspberry and Lemon Juice 111
23. Basil and Celery Smoothie 113
24. Burdock Root and Ginger Soup with Basil 115

TREATING DIGESTIVE ISSUES AND LIVER DETOX 117
Common Digestive Problems and Their Causes 118
Dr. Sebi's Detoxification Methods 120
Alkaline Foods for Digestive Health 121
Liver Cleansing Protocols 122
4 Recipes for Healing Digestive Issues 125
25. Ginger and Fennel Tea 125
26. Papaya and Mango Smoothie 127
27. Chamomile and Peppermint Infusion 129
28. Aloe Vera and Cucumber Juice 131
4 Recipes for Liver Problems 133
29. Dandelion Root Tea 133
30. Liver-Supporting Kale and Walnut Smoothie 135
31. Zucchini and Lemon Salad 137
32. Beet and Carrot Liver Cleanse Juice 139

PROMOTING HAIR GROWTH AND TREATING HAIR LOSS 141
Causes of Hair Loss 143
Dr. Sebi's Herbal Remedies for Hair Health 145
Nutritional Tips for Healthy Hair 146
Recipes for Treating Hair Loss 147
33. Scalp Nourishing Hair Mask 148
34. Stimulating Scalp Massage Oil 149
35. Revitalizing Protein Hair Rinse 150

THE IMPORTANCE OF DETOXIFICATION 152
- The Role of Detoxification in Health 153
- Dr. Sebi's Detoxification Methods Explained 155
- Step-by-Step Detox Plans 156

DR. SEBI'S RECOMMENDED LIFESTYLE CHANGES 159
- Stress Management and Mental Health 160
- Importance of Exercise 162
- Sleep and Recovery 163
- Avoiding Environmental Toxins 164

PRACTICAL TIPS AND TRICKS FOR DAILY LIFE 166
- Maintaining a Balanced pH Level 167
- Reading Food Labels 168
- Building a Support System 170

CONCLUSION 172
- Recap of Key Points 172
- Encouragement for Your Healing Journey 173
- Additional Resources and Further Reading 174

APPENDICES 176
- Detailed Herb Glossary 178
- Frequently Asked Questions 179
- Resources for Further Information 180
- Contact Information for Support and Community 181

INTRODUCTION

Welcome to a journey through the healing wisdom of Dr. Sebi, a path that promises to transform your understanding of health and wellness. Dr. Sebi's legacy is not just about the herbal remedies he championed, but about a fundamental shift in how we view our bodies, our health, and the natural world that sustains us. At the heart of this journey is the belief that nature holds the key to our healing and that by aligning our lives with nature's principles, we can overcome a myriad of health challenges. This book is designed to introduce you to the core concepts of Dr. Sebi's teachings, focusing on the power of an alkaline diet, the importance of detoxification, and the use of natural herbs to treat diseases that modern medicine struggles to manage. Whether you're grappling with chronic illness, seeking to improve your general well-being, or simply curious about alternative health practices, you'll find valuable insights and practical advice within these pages. Our exploration is grounded in the understanding that many of you are approaching this topic for the first time, seeking solutions outside the conventional medical system that has left you wanting more. With an open mind and a willingness to embrace a new perspective on health, you're taking the first step towards a more vibrant, healthful life. Dr. Sebi's approach is more than just a diet; it's a lifestyle change that emphasizes the importance of living in harmony with nature's laws. As we delve into the specifics of how to naturally address diseases such as diabetes, high blood pressure, and even more complex conditions like lupus and cancer, remember that this journey is about empowerment. It's about equipping you with the knowledge and tools to take control of your health, using the healing power of nature. So, let's embark on this transformative journey together, with the spirit of curiosity and the goal of unlocking the secrets to a healthier, more fulfilling life.

Preface: Understanding Dr. Sebi's Legacy

Dr. Sebi, born Alfredo Darrington Bowman, was a Honduran herbalist and healer whose approach to health has captivated and helped thousands worldwide. His philosophy was simple yet revolutionary: he believed that a diet consisting solely of natural alkaline plants and herbs could detoxify the body, thereby curing it of a multitude of diseases. Dr. Sebi's legacy is built on the foundation that returning to a "natural state"—where our diets are in harmony with the evolutionary aspects of our biology—can lead to an unparalleled state of health and wellness.

His methodology focused on the alkaline diet, which emphasizes the consumption of plants and herbs that shift the body's pH to a more alkaline state. According to Dr. Sebi, this is crucial for combating the acidity that is often the root cause of many ailments. He argued that diseases cannot survive in an alkaline environment and that by eliminating acidic foods, individuals could heal themselves of conditions that conventional medicine deemed incurable.

Dr. Sebi's treatments and dietary recommendations were not just about food; they were about reawakening an innate connection to the earth and its healing properties. He championed the use of natural, mineral-rich foods and herbs, advocating for a lifestyle that was in sync with nature. His approach was holistic, considering the physical, emotional, and spiritual health of an individual as interconnected and essential to overall well-being.

Despite facing criticism and legal challenges, Dr. Sebi remained steadfast in his beliefs, leaving behind a legacy that continues to inspire those seeking alternative paths to health and healing. His teachings have sparked a movement towards natural living and wellness, encouraging people to look beyond conventional medicine and explore the healing power of nature. As we delve into the specifics of his approach and the treatments he recommended, it's important to remember the core of his message: nature holds the key to our healing, and by aligning ourselves with its wisdom, we can achieve a state of health and vitality that transcends conventional understanding.

The Importance of Natural Healing

The importance of natural healing lies in its ability to work with the body's inherent systems, promoting wellness from the inside out. In a world where conventional medicine often focuses on treating symptoms rather than underlying causes, natural healing methods offer a refreshing alternative that seeks to restore balance and health in a holistic manner. By turning to the earth for remedies—be it through diet, herbal medicine, or lifestyle adjustments—we tap into ancient wisdom that has sustained human health for millennia.

Natural healing emphasizes the prevention of disease as much as the treatment, encouraging practices that support the body's own healing mechanisms. This approach is grounded in the understanding that our bodies are designed to heal themselves, given the right conditions. By nourishing our bodies with alkaline foods, engaging in regular physical activity, ensuring adequate rest, and managing stress, we create an environment conducive to healing and long-term health.

One of the core principles of natural healing is the belief that what we eat has a profound impact on our health. An alkaline diet, rich in fruits, vegetables, nuts, and seeds, helps to reduce inflammation and acidity in the body, conditions often linked to chronic diseases. This way of eating supports the body's natural pH balance, promoting optimal function of all bodily systems.

Herbal medicine, another cornerstone of natural healing, utilizes the potent properties of plants to address a wide range of health issues. From boosting the immune system to improving digestion, herbs offer targeted support without the harsh side effects often associated with pharmaceutical drugs. This is not to dismiss the value of conventional medicine, but to highlight that integrating natural remedies can enhance overall well-being and support the body's healing process.

Moreover, natural healing advocates for a lifestyle that minimizes exposure to toxins—be it through the food we eat, the products we use, or the environment we live in. Detoxification, through methods such as fasting, herbal cleanses, and sauna therapy, plays a crucial role in eliminating accumulated toxins and rejuvenating the body.

In embracing natural healing, we also acknowledge the importance of mental and emotional well-being as integral to physical health. Stress management techniques such as meditation, yoga, and deep breathing exercises are vital tools in maintaining a balanced and healthy life.

For those who have grown disillusioned with the limitations of conventional medicine, or who seek to take a more active role in their health, natural healing offers a path to empowerment. It encourages individuals to listen to their bodies, to connect with nature, and to make informed choices about their health and wellness.

In conclusion, the importance of natural healing cannot be overstated. It represents a holistic approach to health that respects the body's wisdom and capacity for self-healing. By aligning with the principles of natural ealing, we can achieve a state of health that is not merely the absence of disease, but a vibrant, thriving existence.

ABOUT DR. SEBI, THE NATURAL HEALER

Dr. Sebi, born Alfredo Darrington Bowman in Honduras in 1933, emerged as a towering figure in the realm of natural healing and holistic wellness. His journey from a humble beginning to becoming a revered herbalist and natural healer is a testament to his unwavering commitment to advocating for a return to nature to find healing and wellness. Dr. Sebi's philosophy centered around the belief that a clear understanding and respect for the laws of nature were paramount in achieving true health. He posited that diseases could not exist in an alkaline environment and thus, through a diet rich in plant-based, nutrient-dense foods, one could restore their health by detoxifying their body and returning to an alkaline state.

His approach was simple yet revolutionary, advocating for a diet that excluded meat, dairy, and processed foods, focusing instead on what he termed "electric foods." These foods, according to Dr. Sebi, are alkaline-forming and conducive to the body's natural healing processes. He developed a comprehensive list of these foods, along with a line of herbal products aimed at detoxifying the body and restoring health. Dr. Sebi's methodology was not just about diet; it was a holistic approach that encompassed mental, spiritual, and physical well-being, emphasizing the interconnectedness of these aspects in achieving overall health.

Despite facing skepticism and legal challenges, Dr. Sebi remained steadfast in his mission, helping thousands of individuals from around the globe. His legacy includes not just the healing of bodies but the empowering of minds, encouraging a shift towards a more conscious and nature-aligned way of living. His work has inspired a movement that continues to grow, driven by the success stories of those who have embraced his teachings and experienced profound transformations in their health and well-being.

Dr. Sebi's influence extends beyond the realm of natural healing; he has become a symbol of resilience, a beacon of hope for those seeking alternatives to conventional medicine. His teachings encourage individuals to take control of their health and to seek wisdom in the simplicity and power of nature. Through his recommended dietary changes and herbal supplements, many have found relief from chronic conditions that were previously thought to be incurable, underscoring the potential of natural healing practices in addressing complex health issues.

For those embarking on a journey towards better health and wellness, Dr. Sebi's principles offer a foundation built on the understanding that the body is capable of remarkable healing, given the right conditions. His legacy is a reminder that, in a world where health often seems elusive, returning to the basics of nature can unveil the path to true and lasting wellness. As we delve deeper into his teachings, we uncover not just the specifics of his dietary recommendations, but the broader implications of adopting a lifestyle that honors the body's natural rhythms and the healing power of the earth. Dr. Sebi's life and work serve as a guiding light, illuminating the path towards a healthier, more vibrant existence, rooted in the wisdom of nature and the power of simplicity.

Biography of Dr. Sebi

Born in the village of Ilanga, Honduras, in 1933, Dr. Sebi grew up in a world far removed from the one he would come to influence. His early life, marked by modest means and a lack of formal education, did not hint at the healer he would become. However, it was perhaps this very simplicity and closeness to nature that laid the groundwork for his future philosophies and practices. Dr. Sebi's journey into the realm of natural healing began out of personal necessity. Suffering from a range of chronic illnesses, including diabetes, asthma, and obesity, he found little relief in conventional medicine. This led him on a quest that took him across the Americas, seeking knowledge from traditional healers, herbalists, and naturalists.

It was in Mexico where Dr. Sebi's transformation took a pivotal turn. Under the mentorship of a local healer, he embraced a diet entirely derived from plants, which he credited for his miraculous recovery. This experience was the cornerstone of what would later become the Dr. Sebi Cell Food philosophy. Dr. Sebi's approach was not merely about diet; it was a holistic view of health that emphasized the importance of living in harmony with nature's laws. He believed that the root of most diseases lay in the accumulation of toxins and that through detoxification, one's health could be restored.

Despite his lack of formal medical training, Dr. Sebi's work gained attention for its effectiveness, drawing clients from around the globe, including celebrities. His legal battles, particularly the 1988 case in New York where he was charged with practicing medicine without a license, only served to increase his fame. Defending himself successfully by producing a number of patients cured of various diseases, Dr. Sebi's legacy was cemented. He continued to advocate for his methods until his death in 2016, leaving behind a body of knowledge that continues to inspire those seeking alternative paths to wellness. Dr. Sebi's biography is a testament to the power of self-education, belief in nature's healing properties, and the potential within everyone to change their health destiny.

Philosophy and Principles

At the heart of Dr. Sebi's teachings lies a profound respect for the laws of nature, a belief that guides his holistic approach to health and wellness. This philosophy is not just about choosing certain foods over others; it's a comprehensive lifestyle that emphasizes the importance of living in alignment with the natural world. Dr. Sebi argued that the human body is inherently alkaline and that maintaining this state through an alkaline diet is key to preventing disease and achieving optimal health. His principles extend beyond diet, incorporating the importance of mental and spiritual wellbeing as integral components of health. According to Dr. Sebi, true healing occurs when there is harmony between the mind, body, and spirit, with nature serving as the ultimate source of healing energy.

Central to Dr. Sebi's philosophy is the concept of "electric foods." These are natural, plant-based foods that are rich in minerals and create an alkaline environment within the body. Dr. Sebi believed that these foods, which include leafy greens, fruits, nuts, and seeds, are "electric" because they are alive and raise the body's vibrational energy. He meticulously identified and promoted a list of such foods that he argued could detoxify the body at a cellular level, thereby restoring health. This emphasis on electric foods is not just about nutrition; it's a call to reconnect with the earth and its natural rhythms, to choose foods that are grown and harvested sustainably, and to foster a deeper appreciation for the bounty that nature provides.

Dr. Sebi's approach to healing also underscored the importance of detoxification. He advocated for fasting and the use of herbal teas and supplements to cleanse the body of toxins accumulated from processed foods, environmental pollutants, and stress. This process of detoxification, according to Dr. Sebi, is essential for restoring the body's natural alkaline state and facilitating healing. It's a principle that encourages individuals to be mindful of what they consume and how it affects their overall health, advocating for a lifestyle that minimizes exposure to toxins not just in food, but in all aspects of life.

Moreover, Dr. Sebi's principles challenge the conventional medical paradigm, proposing that most diseases stem from the accumulation of mucus in the body, which is exacerbated by acidic foods. His solution—a shift towards an alkaline, mucus-less diet—offers a radical yet simple approach to preventing and reversing disease. This perspective encourages individuals to take control of their health by making informed choices about their diet and lifestyle, empowering them to act as their own healers.

His teachings continue to resonate with many who seek a holistic approach to health, one that honors the interconnectedness of all living things and recognizes the healing power of nature. Through his legacy, Dr. Sebi inspires us to embrace simplicity, to nourish our bodies with natural, electric foods, and to live in a way that is in harmony with the earth.

Key Contributions to Natural Healing

Dr. Sebi's contributions to the realm of natural healing are both profound and transformative, offering a blueprint for wellness that diverges significantly from conventional medical practices. His advocacy for a plant-based diet, rich in alkaline foods, has reshaped the way many think about nutrition, disease prevention, and the healing capabilities of the human body. Central to his contributions is the development of the African Bio-Mineral Balance, a therapeutic approach that replenishes the body with minerals and nutrients it is naturally aligned with, due to their alkaline nature. This method stands as a testament to his belief in the power of natural substances to restore health, challenging the reliance on pharmaceuticals and processed foods.

Dr. Sebi's herbal compounds and dietary guidelines have provided a foundation for detoxifying the body, a crucial step in reversing disease and restoring health. His unique perspective on the cause of disease, attributing it to mucus buildup resulting from an acidic diet (as previously touched upon), has led to the creation of a dietary regimen that supports the body's natural alkaline state. This approach has not only offered hope to those suffering from chronic conditions but also ignited a broader conversation about the impact of diet on overall health.

Moreover, Dr. Sebi's emphasis on electric foods introduces a novel classification of nourishment. These foods, according to him, are endowed with a higher vibrational energy that is essential for the body's cellular rejuvenation and healing. By identifying and promoting the consumption of these foods, he has guided many towards dietary choices that support both physical and energetic well-being.

Another significant contribution is his challenge to the conventional medical paradigm, advocating for self-healing through dietary and lifestyle changes. This empowerment of individuals to take control of their health has fostered a community of people who are more informed about their health choices, skeptical of one-size-fits-all medical solutions, and committed to living in a way that promotes wellness.

Dr. Sebi's influence also extends to his legal battles, which brought his methodologies into the public eye, offering a platform to challenge the status quo and advocate for the legitimacy of natural healing practices. His victory in court is not just a personal triumph, but a victory for alternative medicine, highlighting the potential of natural remedies to stand up to scrutiny and produce tangible health outcomes.

In essence, Dr. Sebi's key contributions to natural healing lie not only in his specific dietary and herbal recommendations but in his broader vision for a healthier humanity. His teachings encourage a reevaluation of the relationship between diet, health, and the environment, advocating for a life that is in harmony with nature's laws. Through his work, Dr. Sebi has left an indelible mark on the field of natural healing, inspiring a movement towards a more holistic and nature-aligned approach to health and wellness.

DR. SEBI'S ALKALINE PLANT-BASED DIET

Dr. Sebi emerged as a beacon of hope for many seeking alternative healing methods outside the conventional medical system. With no formal medical training, his profound understanding of natural herbs and their healing properties catapulted him into the limelight as a self-taught herbalist whose methodologies challenged the very foundations of Western medicine. Dr. Sebi's philosophy was rooted in the simple yet revolutionary concept that diseases could only exist in an acidic environment and that creating an alkaline state within the body could prevent or cure illness. His approach was holistic, emphasizing the need to cleanse the body of toxins, support immune function, and nourish the body with mineral-rich foods.

Central to Dr. Sebi's teachings was the alkaline diet, a regimen that excludes acidic, processed foods and focuses on natural, plant-based ingredients. He identified a list of specific alkaline foods that he believed were conducive to optimal health, including fruits, vegetables, nuts, and seeds that are native to the African genome. Dr. Sebi argued that these foods help maintain the body's natural alkalinity, which can prevent the accumulation of toxins that lead to disease.

Despite facing skepticism and legal challenges, Dr. Sebi's influence grew, with many attesting to the effectiveness of his treatments in addressing chronic conditions that conventional medicine had failed to remedy. His legacy is a testament to the power of natural healing and the potential of the human body to recover and thrive when supported by the right nutrients and a clean environment. Dr. Sebi's work continues to inspire a movement towards natural wellness, encouraging individuals to explore holistic approaches to health that prioritize the body's innate wisdom over pharmaceutical interventions.

The Science Behind the Alkaline Diet

The science behind the alkaline diet is both fascinating and foundational to understanding how we can harness the power of nutrition to support our body's health. At its core, the alkaline diet is based on the premise that the foods we eat can affect the pH balance of our body, which in turn influences our overall health. The human body naturally maintains a slightly alkaline pH level, which is essential for optimal functioning of cells, tissues, and organs. When we consume foods that are acidic, it can disrupt this delicate balance, leading to a host of health issues.

Foods are classified as acidic, neutral, or alkaline based on their potential renal acid load (PRAL) score. This score indicates the amount of acid that is expected to reach the kidneys after the body metabolizes the foods. Alkaline foods, such as most fruits and vegetables, have a negative PRAL score, meaning they can help neutralize acidity in the body. On the other hand, foods like meat, dairy, and processed foods have a positive PRAL score, contributing to acidity.

The alkaline diet encourages the consumption of alkaline-forming foods to help maintain the body's pH balance. This is not about changing the pH of the blood, which the body tightly regulates, but rather influencing the overall pH environment within the body. By doing so, proponents of the alkaline diet argue that we can reduce inflammation, prevent disease, and promote healing.

One of the key benefits of an alkaline diet is its impact on bone health. Research has shown that consuming foods with a high acidic load can lead to a decrease in bone density over time. This is because the body may leach calcium from the bones, an alkaline mineral, to neutralize the excess acid. By adopting an alkaline diet, you can help protect your bones and reduce the risk of osteoporosis.

Additionally, an alkaline diet can support kidney health. The kidneys play a crucial role in filtering out toxins and managing the body's acid-base balance. A diet high in acidic foods can put additional strain on the kidneys, potentially leading to kidney stones or other renal issues. By consuming more alkaline foods, you can help ease the burden on your kidneys, supporting their function and health.

Moreover, an alkaline diet can have a positive effect on cardiovascular health. Studies have suggested that an alkaline diet can help lower blood pressure and reduce the risk of hypertension, a major risk factor for heart disease. The high intake of fruits, vegetables, and other nutrient-rich, alkaline-forming foods can also support healthy cholesterol levels and improve overall heart health.

For those new to the concept, transitioning to an alkaline diet doesn't have to be overwhelming. Start by gradually increasing your intake of alkaline-forming foods while reducing acidic foods. Focus on incorporating a variety of fruits and vegetables, nuts, seeds, and legumes into your diet. Remember, the goal is not to eliminate acidic foods entirely but to create a more balanced and health-supportive diet.

In embracing the alkaline diet, you're not just changing what you eat; you're adopting a holistic approach to health that considers the impact of food on your body's natural balance. While the alkaline diet is not a cure-all, it offers a powerful tool for enhancing your health and well-being, grounded in the understanding of the body's natural processes and the healing power of food.

Benefits of an Alkaline Diet

Adopting an alkaline diet brings a multitude of health benefits, directly impacting your energy levels, digestion, and even your mood. By focusing on alkaline-forming foods, you're essentially fueling your body with the optimal nutrients it needs to thrive. One of the immediate benefits many report is a significant boost in energy and clarity of mind. This isn't surprising, considering that alkaline foods, rich in vitamins and minerals, support mitochondrial function, the powerhouse of our cells, thereby enhancing energy production.

Digestive health also sees remarkable improvement on an alkaline diet. Alkaline foods, being high in fiber, naturally aid in digestion and help to maintain a healthy gut flora. This can lead to reduced bloating, improved bowel movements, and a decrease in gastrointestinal discomfort. Moreover, an alkaline environment in the gut discourages the growth of harmful bacteria and encourages the presence of beneficial microbes, contributing to overall gut health.

Another notable benefit is the positive effect on skin health. Alkaline foods are loaded with antioxidants and hydration, which can help to flush out toxins, leading to clearer, more radiant skin. The high content of antioxidants in these foods fights free radicals, reducing inflammation and preventing premature aging.

Weight management is another area where the alkaline diet shines. By emphasizing whole foods and minimizing processed foods, sugars, and fats, which are typically acidic, the diet naturally promotes a healthy weight. The high fiber content in alkaline-forming foods also means you feel fuller longer, reducing the likelihood of overeating and snacking on unhealthy options.

Lastly, the alkaline diet supports overall immune function. The diet's emphasis on fruits, vegetables, nuts, and seeds ensures that you're getting a wide range of essential nutrients and antioxidants that bolster the immune system. A strong immune system is better equipped to fend off infections and diseases, keeping you healthier in the long run.

Incorporating more alkaline foods into your diet is a simple yet powerful way to enhance your health and well-being. Whether you're looking to boost your energy, improve digestion, or support your immune system, the alkaline diet offers a natural, holistic approach to achieving optimal health.

Essential Alkaline Foods

Embarking on an alkaline diet involves incorporating a variety of essential alkaline foods that are not only nutritious, but also promote an alkaline environment within your body. These foods help balance the body's pH level, supporting overall health and preventing various diseases. Fruits and vegetables are the cornerstone of any alkaline diet, offering a rich source of minerals, vitamins, and antioxidants that help neutralize acidic waste and enhance your body's natural healing abilities.

Leafy greens such as kale and Swiss chard are particularly beneficial, packed with chlorophyll, which has a powerful alkalizing effect on the body. These greens are versatile and can be enjoyed in salads, smoothies, or as a steamed side dish. Avocados, a source of healthy fats, fiber, and essential nutrients, also play a significant role in maintaining an alkaline state. They can be added to almost any meal, providing creaminess and flavor.

Cucumbers and celery are known for their high water content and alkalizing properties, making them perfect for hydration and as a crunchy snack or salad addition.

Alkaline fruits like lemons, limes, and grapefruits may seem acidic, but they actually have an alkalizing effect once digested. Starting your day with a glass of lemon water can kickstart digestion and help balance your pH levels. Melons and berries are also excellent choices, providing hydration, antioxidants, and a variety of vitamins.

Nuts and seeds, such as hemp seeds, raw sesame seeds, and walnuts, are alkaline-forming and a great source of omega-3 fatty acids, protein, and fiber. Soaking nuts and seeds overnight can enhance their nutritional value and make them easier to digest. Quinoa and buckwheat are alkaline grains that offer a high-protein alternative to traditional wheat or rice, suitable for those looking to maintain an alkaline diet.

Herbal teas, particularly those made from ginger, dandelion, and green tea, support alkalinity and offer various health benefits, including improved digestion and detoxification. Incorporating these essential alkaline foods into your diet can lead to improved energy levels, better digestion, and a stronger immune system, helping you to feel your best.

Remember, the goal of an alkaline diet is not to eliminate all acidic foods, but to achieve a balance that supports your body's natural pH level. By focusing on whole, unprocessed foods and minimizing the intake of sugar, caffeine, and processed foods, you can create a diet that not only supports alkalinity but also promotes overall health and well-being.

Tips for Maintaining an Alkaline Lifestyle

Maintaining an alkaline lifestyle goes beyond just adjusting your diet; it encompasses a holistic approach to living that promotes health and well-being. To successfully integrate this lifestyle, consider incorporating these practical tips into your daily routine. First and foremost, hydration is key. Drinking plenty of alkaline water, ideally with a pH level above 7, helps flush toxins from the body and maintain a balanced internal environment. Aim for at least eight 8-ounce glasses of water daily, and consider adding a slice of lemon or lime to enhance its alkalizing effect.

Next, focus on mindful eating habits. Prioritize fresh, whole foods over processed items, and take the time to enjoy your meals without distractions. This not only aids digestion, but also helps you appreciate the natural flavors of alkaline-forming foods. Incorporating a wide variety of fruits and vegetables into your meals ensures you receive a broad spectrum of nutrients and antioxidants, supporting overall health.

Exercise is another cornerstone of an alkaline lifestyle. Regular physical activity, whether it's walking, yoga, or any form of exercise you enjoy, helps reduce stress, improve circulation, and boost mood. Exercise also enhances the body's natural detoxification processes, promoting an alkaline state.

Stress management is crucial in maintaining an alkaline lifestyle. High stress levels can lead to an acidic internal environment, negating the benefits of an alkaline diet. Incorporate stress-reducing practices such as meditation, deep breathing exercises, or spending time in nature into your daily routine to help maintain your body's alkalinity.

Sleep plays a vital role in health and well-being, including the maintenance of an alkaline state. Ensure you get adequate, quality sleep each night to support your body's healing and regeneration processes. Establishing a calming bedtime routine can improve sleep quality and help your body recover from the day's activities.

Limiting the intake of acidic substances such as caffeine, alcohol, and tobacco is essential for maintaining an alkaline lifestyle. These substances can disrupt the body's pH balance and overall health. Instead, opt for herbal teas and natural, non-alcoholic beverages that support alkalinity.

Finally, fostering a positive mindset and emotional well-being is an often-overlooked aspect of an alkaline lifestyle. Positive thoughts and emotions can influence physical health, promoting a balanced and harmonious state of being. Engage in activities that bring you joy, spend time with loved ones, and practice gratitude to enhance your mental and emotional health.

By integrating these tips into your life, you can maintain an alkaline lifestyle that supports your health and well-being. Remember, the goal is not perfection but progress. Making small, sustainable changes over time can lead to significant improvements in your health and quality of life.

Common Mistakes to Avoid

Embarking on an alkaline lifestyle can be a transformative journey toward better health and well-being, but it's not without its pitfalls. One common mistake is the overconsumption of high-sugar fruits. While fruits are an essential part of an alkaline diet, it's important to balance your intake with a variety of vegetables, especially leafy greens, to avoid excessive sugar intake which can counteract the benefits of alkalinity.

Another pitfall is neglecting hydration. Drinking enough water is crucial for flushing toxins from the body and maintaining alkaline balance. However, simply drinking water isn't enough; ensuring it's alkaline water with a pH level above 7 (as mentioned in the previous section) can further support your body's pH balance. Neglecting this aspect can slow down the detoxification process and diminish the diet's effectiveness.

Many beginners mistakenly believe that adopting an alkaline lifestyle means they must strictly avoid all acidic foods. This is not the case. Balance is key. Completely eliminating acidic foods is not only unrealistic but also unnecessary. The goal is to achieve a healthy balance where alkaline-forming foods predominate without completely excluding the nutritional benefits of certain acidic foods.

Failing to plan meals is another common error that can derail your efforts. Without proper planning, it's easy to fall back on processed foods or meals that don't align with an alkaline diet. Taking the time to plan and prepare alkaline-rich meals ensures you have the right foods on hand when hunger strikes, making it easier to stick to your goals.

Overlooking the importance of organic produce is another oversight. Non-organic fruits and vegetables can contain pesticides and chemicals that increase the body's toxic load, working against the alkaline diet's detoxifying effects. Whenever possible, choose organic to reduce exposure to these harmful substances.

Some individuals also underestimate the importance of a holistic approach, focusing solely on diet while neglecting other aspects of a healthy lifestyle that support alkalinity, such as stress management, regular exercise, and adequate sleep. These elements are integral to maintaining an alkaline state and should not be overlooked.

Ignoring the body's signals is a critical mistake. Everyone's body responds differently to dietary changes. What works for one person may not work for another. Paying attention to how your body reacts to different foods and adjusting your diet accordingly is essential for finding the right balance that works for you.

Lastly, expecting immediate results can lead to disappointment. Transitioning to an alkaline lifestyle is a process that requires time and patience. Immediate changes in health and well-being may not be evident, but with consistency, the long-term benefits can be significant.

Avoiding these common mistakes can help ensure a smoother transition to an alkaline lifestyle, paving the way for improved health and vitality. Remember, the journey to better health is a marathon, not a sprint, and small, consistent changes can lead to lasting benefits.

DEALING WITH HERPES AND HIV

Herpes and HIV, two viral infections that have challenged the medical community for decades, can significantly impact the quality of life. Dr. Sebi's approach to these conditions emphasizes the body's inherent ability to heal itself through natural, holistic methods. By focusing on immune-boosting foods and herbs, alongside detailed detoxification processes, individuals can take proactive steps towards managing symptoms and improving their overall health.

Understanding herpes and HIV begins with recognizing the viral nature of these conditions and their effects on the body. Herpes simplex virus (HSV) can cause both oral and genital herpes, leading to blisters and sores. Human Immunodeficiency Virus (HIV), on the other hand, attacks the immune system, progressively weakening it and, if left untreated, can lead to Acquired Immunodeficiency Syndrome (AIDS). Dr. Sebi's natural treatment methods for these viruses involve a strict dietary regimen, focused on alkaline foods that reduce acidity in the body, creating an environment less conducive to viral replication.

Immune-boosting foods and herbs are central to Dr. Sebi's protocol. Foods high in minerals, vitamins, and antioxidants are recommended to strengthen the immune system. These include leafy greens, nuts, seeds, and fruits like berries and melons. Herbs such as elderberry and burdock root are known for their immune-enhancing properties and are suggested for daily consumption.

The detailed detoxification processes outlined by Dr. Sebi aim to cleanse the body of toxins and waste, further supporting immune function. This involves fasting, herbal teas, and the use of specific supplements to aid in the elimination of toxins. Detoxification is considered a crucial step in creating an optimal internal environment for healing and recovery.

For those seeking practical applications of Dr. Sebi's teachings, five recipes for healing herpes and HIV are provided, each designed to incorporate immune-boosting ingredients and alkaline foods. These recipes include an herbal antiviral tea, blending lemon balm, peppermint, and elderberry for their antiviral properties; an alkaline detox soup, featuring alkaline vegetables and sea moss; an antioxidant-rich salad, loaded with leafy greens, nuts, and seeds; and a healing herbal infusion, made with burdock root and dandelion to support liver function and detoxification.

By adhering to Dr. Sebi's guidelines, individuals dealing with herpes and HIV can empower themselves to take control of their health through natural, holistic means. It's important to remember that while these methods can offer significant benefits, they should complement, not replace, the advice and treatment plans provided by healthcare professionals. The journey towards health and wellness is personal and multifaceted, encompassing diet, lifestyle, and mental well-being. Through dedication to Dr. Sebi's principles, those affected by herpes and HIV can pursue a path towards improved health and vitality, embracing the power of nature's healing capabilities.

Understanding Herpes and HIV

Herpes and HIV are two viral infections that have significant impacts on health, each with its own set of challenges and misconceptions. Herpes, caused by the herpes simplex virus (HSV), manifests primarily as sores on the mouth or genitals, depending on whether it's HSV-1 or HSV-2. It's a common infection, with many people showing no symptoms yet capable of transmitting the virus to others. On the other hand, HIV, the Human Immunodeficiency Virus, attacks the immune system, specifically the CD4 cells, making the body more vulnerable to infections and diseases. Without treatment, HIV can progress to AIDS, the last stage of HIV infection, where the immune system is severely damaged.

Both viruses are highly stigmatized, often leading to significant emotional and psychological distress for those diagnosed. Understanding these conditions is the first step toward demystifying them and promoting a more compassionate and informed approach to health.

Herpes simplex virus is highly contagious and can be transmitted through direct contact with an infected person's skin or mucous membranes. This means that kissing, sexual contact, and even sharing utensils or lip balm with someone who has herpes can spread the virus. Once infected, the virus remains in the body for life, lying dormant in nerve cells and occasionally causing outbreaks of sores.

HIV is transmitted through contact with infected blood, semen, vaginal fluids, or breast milk. The most common ways HIV is spread are through unprotected sex, sharing needles for drug use, and from mother to child during birth or breastfeeding. Unlike herpes, HIV does not remain dormant; it continuously attacks the immune system. Antiretroviral therapy (ART) can effectively manage HIV, allowing individuals to live long, healthy lives with the virus. ART works by reducing the amount of virus in the body, which helps the immune system recover and reduces the risk of transmitting the virus to others.

Prevention of both herpes and HIV focuses on avoiding exposure to the viruses. For herpes, this means avoiding contact with the sores of an infected person and using barrier methods, like condoms, during sexual activity. For HIV, prevention also includes the use of condoms, as well as pre-exposure prophylaxis (PrEP), a medication taken by HIV-negative individuals to reduce the risk of infection if exposed to the virus.

The emotional and social implications of living with herpes or HIV can be profound. The stigma surrounding these infections can lead to feelings of shame, isolation, and depression. It's crucial for individuals diagnosed with either condition to seek support, whether through counseling, support groups, or trusted friends and family. Education plays a vital role in breaking down the stigma, as understanding the facts about these viruses can help dispel myths and promote empathy.

In managing herpes and HIV, a holistic approach that includes both medical treatment and lifestyle adjustments can be beneficial. Stress management, a healthy diet, and regular exercise can help strengthen the immune system and improve overall well-being. For those living with HIV, adhering to ART is essential for managing the virus and maintaining health.

In conclusion, herpes and HIV are two conditions that, while challenging, can be managed with proper care and treatment. Understanding these viruses is key to prevention, effective management, and reducing the stigma that affects those living with them. By fostering a supportive and informed community, we can help improve the lives of those affected by herpes and HIV.

Dr. Sebi's Natural Treatment Methods

Dr. Sebi's natural treatment methods revolve around the core principle that a properly nourished body is capable of healing itself from within. His approach, as we have touched on, is deeply rooted in the belief that diseases cannot thrive in an alkaline environment, hence his emphasis on transitioning to an alkaline diet. This diet focuses on consuming foods that transform the body's pH level from acidic to alkaline, which is conducive to optimal health.

Beyond diet, Dr. Sebi advocated for the use of specific herbs to cleanse the body's organs and remove toxins that contribute to disease. His herbal compounds were designed to cleanse the body's cells by eliminating deeply rooted toxins, thereby restoring the body to its natural state of health and vitality. For instance, his detox teas and supplements target the liver, kidneys, blood, and lymphatic system for a comprehensive detoxification.

Dr. Sebi also stressed the importance of hydration, recommending the consumption of a gallon of natural spring water daily to assist in flushing out toxins and maintaining cellular hydration. He believed that proper hydration is key to maintaining an alkaline environment within the body.

Another pillar of Dr. Sebi's treatment methods is fasting. Fasting is utilized as a means to give the digestive system a break, allowing the body to focus its energy on healing. During fasting, the consumption of his recommended herbal teas and water is encouraged to aid in the detoxification process.

Dr. Sebi's approach is holistic, not only addressing the physical aspects of health, but also emphasizing the importance of mental and emotional well-being. He advocated for practices such as meditation and spending time in nature to reduce stress and promote a balanced state of mind, which he considered essential for healing.

For those new to Dr. Sebi's methods, starting with a gradual shift towards an alkaline diet, incorporating specific herbs for detoxification, staying hydrated, and practicing fasting and stress-reduction techniques can be transformative. It's about making lifestyle changes that align with natural principles of health and well-being. Dr. Sebi's legacy continues to inspire individuals seeking to heal naturally, emphasizing that with the right nourishment and care, the body has an innate ability to heal itself.

Immune-Boosting Foods and Herbs

Boosting your immune system is a key component of maintaining health and warding off diseases, and nature has provided us with an abundance of foods and herbs that can help strengthen our body's defenses. Incorporating immune-boosting foods and herbs into your diet is a simple yet effective way to enhance your body's ability to fight infections and diseases. These natural remedies are packed with essential nutrients and compounds that support immune function, promote health, and can be easily integrated into your daily routine.

Foods rich in vitamin C, such as Seville or sour oranges, strawberries, and bell peppers (but not green bell peppers) are well-known for their immune-boosting properties. Vitamin C is a powerful antioxidant that helps protect the body against infection and supports the function of various immune cells. It also plays a crucial role in the repair and regeneration of tissues, making it essential for overall health and well-being.

Another key nutrient for immune health is vitamin D, which can be found in foods like mushrooms (although one should avoid Shitake mushrooms), as well as through exposure to sunlight. Vitamin D is critical for the activation of immune system defenses, and low levels have been associated with an increased risk of infection.

Zinc is a mineral that is vital for immune function and can be found in foods such as lentils and chickpeas. Zinc helps the immune system fight off invading bacteria and viruses, and a deficiency in this nutrient can lead to a weakened immune response.

In addition to these nutrients, there are several herbs known for their immune-enhancing properties.

A particularly powerful herb is elderberry, which is rich in antioxidants and vitamins that can boost the immune system. Elderberry has antiviral properties and has been shown to reduce the severity and duration of cold and flu symptoms.

Ginger is also excellent for immune health. Ginger has anti-inflammatory and antioxidative properties, helping to reduce inflammation and support the immune system.

Incorporating these immune-boosting foods and herbs into your diet can be simple and delicious. Start your day with a smoothie made with fruits high in vitamin C, add ginger to your cooking, and consider taking herbal supplements like elderberry during cold and flu season.

Remember, while these foods and herbs can support your immune system, they are not a substitute for a healthy lifestyle. Regular exercise, adequate sleep, stress management, and a balanced diet are all crucial for maintaining optimal immune function and overall health. By combining these lifestyle practices with the power of immune-boosting foods and herbs, you can help protect yourself against infections and diseases and promote long-term well-being.

Detailed Detoxification Processes

Detoxification is a natural process your body undertakes to neutralize or eliminate toxins through the major organs such as the liver, kidneys, intestines, lungs, lymphatic system, and skin. However, due to increased exposure to pollutants, chemicals, and unhealthy diets, assisting your body in this detoxification process has become more crucial than ever. Dr. Sebi's detoxification processes emphasize the importance of aiding the body in this natural cleansing effort through diet, fasting, and the use of specific herbs.

The first step in the detoxification process is to reduce the intake of toxins. This means adopting an alkaline diet that excludes processed foods, dairy, meat, and sugar while increasing the intake of whole, natural foods like fruits, vegetables, and whole grains that are organic and non-GMO whenever possible. These foods are less taxing on the body's detoxification systems and provide the necessary nutrients and antioxidants that support cleansing.

Fasting is another cornerstone of Dr. Sebi's detoxification process, as we have made clear. By abstaining from eating for certain periods, you give your digestive system a break, allowing your body to focus its energy on healing and detoxification. During a fast, it is recommended to drink plenty of alkaline water and herbal teas to help flush toxins from the body. A simple way to start is with intermittent fasting, gradually increasing the fasting window as your body adjusts.

Herbal teas play a significant role in the detoxification process. Herbs such as burdock root, dandelion, and sarsaparilla are known for their powerful cleansing properties. These herbs help purify the blood, cleanse the liver, and aid the kidneys in filtering toxins. Drinking herbal teas daily can significantly enhance the body's ability to detoxify naturally.

The liver, being the primary organ responsible for detoxification, requires specific attention. Herbs like milk thistle and dandelion support liver health and function. Incorporating these herbs into your diet through teas or supplements can help boost your liver's ability to detoxify the blood.

The lymphatic system, another critical component of the body's detoxification process, benefits from hydration, exercise, and dry brushing. Staying hydrated ensures that lymph fluid can flow freely, while exercise stimulates lymphatic circulation. Dry brushing, performed with a natural bristle brush on dry skin before showering, helps stimulate the lymphatic system and remove dead skin cells, further aiding in detoxification.

Finally, it's essential to support your kidneys, which filter waste and excess fluids from the blood. Consuming foods high in antioxidants and low in salt, like blueberries, and beets, can help maintain kidney health. Additionally, herbs such as nettle are beneficial for kidney cleansing and can be consumed as teas.

In summary, Dr. Sebi's detailed detoxification processes focus on reducing toxin intake, fasting, consuming an alkaline diet rich in whole foods, and using specific herbs to support the body's natural detoxification organs. By following these guidelines, you can assist your body in its natural cleansing processes, leading to improved health and vitality. Remember, detoxification is a continuous process and incorporating these practices into your lifestyle can help maintain your body's natural balance and wellness.

4 Recipes for Healing Herpes and HIV

1. Herbal Antiviral Tea

Beneficial effects

This Herbal Antiviral Tea is designed to strengthen the immune system and combat viral infections. The selected herbs are known for their antiviral properties, making this tea an excellent choice for individuals looking to naturally support their body's defense against conditions like herpes and HIV. Regular consumption can help reduce inflammation, boost immune function, and provide antiviral support.

Portions	Preparation time	Cooking time
Makes about 2 servings	10 minutes	15 minutes

Ingredients

- 1 tablespoon of dried elderberry
- 1 teaspoon of dried lemon balm
- 1/2 teaspoon of dried ginger root
- 4 cups of water

Instructions

1. Combine the dried elderberry, echinacea, lemon balm, and ginger root in a medium-sized pot.
2. Add 4 cups of water to the pot and bring the mixture to a boil over high heat.
3. Once boiling, reduce the heat to low and let the tea simmer for about 15 minutes. This allows the water to become infused with the herbs' properties.
4. After simmering, remove the pot from the heat and let the tea cool slightly for a few minutes.
5. Strain the tea into cups or a large container, removing all the solid herb pieces.

6. Serve the tea warm for immediate use, or allow it to cool completely for chilled tea.

Variations

- For a citrus twist, add a slice of lemon or a few drops of lemon juice to each cup before serving.

- Incorporate a cinnamon stick during the simmering process for added flavor and potential blood sugar regulation benefits.

Storage tips

Store any leftover tea in the refrigerator in a sealed container for up to 3 days. Reheat gently on the stove or enjoy cold.

Tips for allergens

Individuals with allergies to any of the herbs should omit them from the recipe or substitute with another herb with similar benefits.

Scientific references

- "Antiviral effects of elderberry juice and extract" in the *Journal of Medicinal Food* highlights elderberry's potential against viral infections.

- "Lemon balm (Melissa officinalis L.) – an overview of its potential in preventing and treating cancer and viral infections" in the *Journal of Nutrition & Food Sciences* outlines lemon balm's antiviral effects.

2. Immune-Boosting Smoothie

Beneficial effects

This Immune-Boosting Smoothie is loaded with essential vitamins, minerals, and antioxidants to bolster the immune system, aiding the body in fighting infections effectively. Ingredients like ginger provide anti-inflammatory benefits, while key lime offers a potent dose of Vitamin C, vital for immune functionality. Callaloo is used as an alternative to spinach, rich in iron and beta-carotene, which are crucial for immune health. Integrating this smoothie into your diet offers a tasty way to boost your body's defenses.

Portions	Preparation time
2 servings	10 minutes

Ingredients

- 1 cup of callaloo, fresh
- 1/2 cup of orange juice (preferably freshly squeezed)
- 1 banana, ripe
- 1/2 cup of frozen mixed berries (such as blueberries, strawberries, and raspberries)
- 1/2 inch piece of ginger, peeled and minced
- 1 tablespoon of agave syrup (optional, for sweetness)
- 1/2 cup of water for desired consistency

Instructions

1. Start by washing the callaloo leaves thoroughly under running water.
2. Peel the banana and cut it into chunks.
3. Take the ginger piece and mince it finely to ensure it blends well into the smoothie.
4. In a blender, combine the callaloo, orange juice, banana chunks, frozen mixed berries, minced ginger.
5. Add agave syrup if you prefer a sweeter taste.
6. Pour in half a cup of water to achieve your desired smoothie consistency.
7. Blend on high speed until all the ingredients are thoroughly mixed and the smoothie has a smooth, creamy texture.

8. Taste and adjust the sweetness if necessary by adding a little more agave syrup.

9. Serve immediately for the best flavor and nutrient retention.

Variations

- For an extra immune boost, add a tablespoon of hemp seeds to the smoothie before blending.

- If you're not a fan of banana, you can substitute it with avocado for creaminess and healthy fats.

- To increase the protein content, add a scoop of your favorite plant-based protein powder.

Storage tips

This smoothie is best enjoyed fresh, but if you need to store it, keep it in an airtight container in the refrigerator for up to 24 hours. Give it a good stir or shake before drinking, as separation may occur.

Tips for allergens

For those who are allergic to nuts omit using them.

Scientific references

- Carr, A.C., Maggini, S. (2017). *Vitamin C and Immune Function. Nutrients*, 9(11), 1211. This study highlights the importance of Vitamin C in immune system function and its role in preventing and treating respiratory and systemic infections.

3. Alkaline Detox Soup

Beneficial effects

This Alkaline Detox Soup is designed to cleanse your body, promote better digestion, and support overall health by creating an alkaline environment in your body. Alkaline diets are believed to help reduce inflammation, boost energy levels, and support the immune system by balancing the body's pH levels. The ingredients in this soup are carefully selected for their alkaline properties and detoxifying effects.

Portions	Preparation time	Cooking time
4 servings	15 minutes	30 minutes

Ingredients

- 1 tablespoon coconut oil
- 1 medium onion, chopped
- 1 small piece of ginger, grated
- 2 cups kale, chopped
- 1 medium zucchini, sliced
- 4 cups vegetable broth (alkaline-friendly, low sodium)
- 1/2 teaspoon sea salt (optional)
- 1/4 teaspoon cayenne pepper
- 1 tablespoon lemon juice

Instructions

1. Heat the coconut oil in a large pot over medium heat. Add the chopped onion and grated ginger. Sauté for about 5 minutes, or until the onions are translucent.
2. Add the chopped kale and sliced zucchini to the pot. Stir well to combine with the onion mixture.
3. Pour the vegetable broth into the pot. Bring the mixture to a boil, then reduce the heat to low and simmer for about 20 minutes, or until the vegetables are tender.
4. Season the soup with sea salt (optional) and cayenne pepper to taste. Add the lemon juice. Stir well.

5. Remove the pot from the heat. Use an immersion blender to blend the soup directly in the pot until smooth. Alternatively, you can blend the soup in batches using a regular blender.

6. Serve the soup warm. Enjoy your alkaline detox soup!

Variations

- For a protein boost, add cooked quinoa or chickpeas to the soup.
- Feel free to include other alkaline vegetables such as avocado or cucumber.
- For a spicy kick, add diced habanero.

Storage tips

Store any leftover soup in an airtight container in the refrigerator for up to 3 days. Reheat on the stove or in the microwave when ready to serve.

Tips for allergens

- For those with coconut allergies, avocado oil can be used as a substitute for coconut oil.
- Ensure the vegetable broth is gluten-free if necessary.

Scientific references

Studies have shown that diets focusing on alkaline foods can help reduce inflammation and the risk of chronic diseases. For example, a review published in the *Journal of Environmental and Public Health* highlights the potential benefits of an alkaline diet in reducing morbidity and mortality from chronic diseases.

4. Antioxidant-Rich Salad

Beneficial effects

This Antioxidant-Rich Salad is a powerhouse of nutrients, designed to boost your immune system and fight off infections. Antioxidants are crucial for maintaining health and preventing diseases, as they protect your body from harmful free radicals that can lead to chronic conditions like heart disease and cancer. The ingredients in this salad are carefully selected to provide a high dose of vitamins, minerals, and antioxidants, promoting overall well-being and supporting the body's natural healing processes.

Portions	Preparation time
4 servings	15 minutes

Ingredients

- 2 cups of fresh callaloo leaves
- 1 cup of sliced strawberries
- 1/2 cup of blueberries
- 1/2 cup of walnuts, roughly chopped
- 1 avocado, sliced
- 1/4 cup of red onion, thinly sliced
- For the dressing:
- 1/4 cup of extra virgin olive oil
- 2 tablespoons of balsamic vinegar
- 1 teaspoon of or agave syrup
- Salt to taste

Instructions

1. In a large salad bowl, combine the callaloo leaves, sliced strawberries, blueberries, and chopped walnuts.
2. Add the sliced avocado, and red onion to the bowl.
3. In a small bowl, whisk together the extra virgin olive oil, balsamic vinegar, agave syrup, and a pinch of salt until well combined.
4. Drizzle the dressing over the salad and gently toss to ensure all the ingredients are evenly coated.

5. Serve immediately for the freshest taste and maximum nutritional benefits.

Variations

- Swap out the berries for other antioxidant-rich fruits like pomegranate seeds or sliced oranges.
- Use lettuce instead of callaloo for a variety of textures and flavors.
- For a nut-free version, substitute hemp or raw sesame seeds for the walnuts.

Storage tips

This salad is best enjoyed fresh. However, if you need to store it, keep the dressing separate and refrigerate the salad and dressing in airtight containers. Consume within 24 hours for optimal freshness.

Tips for allergens

- For a dairy-free version, omit the feta cheese or use a dairy-free cheese alternative.
- Ensure the nuts used are suitable for those with nut allergies, or use seeds as a safe alternative.

Scientific references

- "Antioxidants in fruits and vegetables: the millennium's health," *International Journal of Food Science & Technology*, highlighting the importance of antioxidants from natural sources in maintaining health and preventing disease.
- "Blueberries, cardiovascular health, and cancer prevention: A review of the current evidence," *American Journal of Clinical Nutrition*, discussing the specific benefits of blueberries, one of the ingredients in this salad.

REVERSING DIABETES NATURALLY

Reversing diabetes naturally is a journey that begins with understanding the root causes of the disease and how lifestyle and dietary choices can significantly impact blood sugar levels and overall health. Diabetes, particularly type 2, is often linked to poor dietary habits, lack of physical activity, and excess weight, which can lead to insulin resistance. This is where the body's cells don't respond effectively to insulin, a hormone that regulates blood sugar levels. Dr. Sebi's approach to combating diabetes focuses on transitioning to an alkaline diet, rich in plant-based, whole foods that naturally help to reduce blood sugar levels and improve insulin sensitivity.

An alkaline diet emphasizes the consumption of fruits, vegetables, nuts, and seeds that are low in sugar and high in nutrients. These foods work by reducing acidity in the body, which Dr. Sebi believed was a major contributor to disease formation, including diabetes. By adopting an alkaline diet, individuals can help their body maintain a healthy pH balance, which supports insulin function and can lead to a natural reversal of diabetes symptoms. Key components of this diet include leafy greens, such as kale and callaloo, which are high in magnesium, a mineral that plays a crucial role in insulin function. Avocados and quinoa are also excellent choices, providing healthy fats, fiber, and protein, which can help manage blood sugar levels.

In addition to dietary changes, Dr. Sebi recommended the use of specific herbs to support the body's healing process. Herbs like burdock root, cinnamon, and fenugreek have been shown to have blood sugar-lowering effects. These herbs can be incorporated into the diet in various forms, such as teas, capsules, or added to foods. For example, cinnamon can be sprinkled on oatmeal or added to smoothies, while fenugreek seeds can be soaked overnight and consumed in the morning to help stabilize blood sugar levels.

Hydration plays a vital role in managing diabetes, as it helps to flush toxins from the body and supports kidney function. Dr. Sebi advocated for the consumption of spring water, which is naturally alkaline, to aid in maintaining the body's pH balance. Drinking adequate amounts of water throughout the day can also help to prevent dehydration, which can affect blood sugar levels.

Physical activity is another crucial aspect of reversing diabetes naturally. Regular exercise helps to improve insulin sensitivity, making it easier for the body to regulate blood sugar levels. It also aids in weight management, which is important for reducing the risk of developing type 2 diabetes or managing the condition if already diagnosed. Dr. Sebi encouraged activities that connect the body with nature, such as walking, gardening, or yoga, as these not only provide physical benefits but also help to reduce stress and promote mental well-being.

It's important to note that while adopting an alkaline diet and making lifestyle changes can have significant benefits for individuals with diabetes, these should be approached gradually and under the guidance of a healthcare professional, especially for those already on medication for diabetes. Monitoring blood sugar levels and adjusting dietary and lifestyle changes as needed is essential for safely managing the condition.

By understanding the principles behind Dr. Sebi's approach to reversing diabetes naturally, individuals can embark on a journey towards restoring their health and vitality. Through a combination of dietary changes, herbal supplements, adequate hydration, and physical activity, it's possible to support the body's healing process and improve diabetes symptoms. As we delve deeper into the specifics of the alkaline diet and how to implement these changes in the next part, remember that each step taken is a step closer to achieving better health and well-being.

Embracing the alkaline diet and incorporating physical activity into daily routines lays a solid foundation for reversing diabetes naturally. Equally important is understanding the role of stress management and its impact on blood sugar levels. Chronic stress can lead to elevated cortisol levels, which in turn can increase blood glucose levels. Incorporating stress-reduction techniques such as meditation, deep breathing exercises, and spending time in nature can help maintain a balanced state of mind, contributing to overall health and the stabilization of blood sugar levels.

Another aspect of Dr. Sebi's holistic approach to reversing diabetes involves paying close attention to sleep patterns. Adequate sleep is crucial for the body's healing process, and lack of sleep can disrupt hormonal balance, including insulin sensitivity. Establishing a regular sleep schedule and creating a restful environment free from electronic devices and other distractions can enhance sleep quality, thereby supporting the body's natural ability to regulate blood sugar levels.

In addition to these lifestyle changes, it's essential to monitor blood sugar levels regularly. This not only helps in assessing the effectiveness of the adopted changes but also in making necessary adjustments to the diet or lifestyle to better manage diabetes. Keeping a food and activity journal can be a useful tool in identifying patterns and triggers that affect blood sugar levels, enabling more informed decisions about daily choices.

The power of community and support cannot be overstated in the journey to reverse diabetes naturally. Joining support groups, whether online or in-person, can provide motivation, encouragement, and valuable information from others who are on a similar path. Sharing experiences and tips can be incredibly empowering and can help individuals feel less isolated in their health journey.

Finally, it's important to remember that reversing diabetes naturally is a gradual process that requires patience, commitment, and consistency. Making small, incremental changes to diet and lifestyle can lead to significant improvements in health over time. It's not about perfection but about making better choices each day that support the body's healing process.

By adopting Dr. Sebi's holistic approach to health, which includes an alkaline diet, regular physical activity, stress management, adequate sleep, and community support, individuals can take control of their diabetes and embark on a path toward improved health and vitality. This journey is not only about managing blood sugar levels but also about embracing a lifestyle that promotes overall well-being. With each step taken, individuals can feel empowered knowing they are nourishing their body, mind, and spirit in a way that aligns with nature's wisdom and the body's innate ability to heal itself.

Understanding Diabetes and Its Causes

Diabetes is a condition that affects the way your body processes blood sugar, or glucose, which is a vital source of energy for the cells that make up your muscles and tissues, as well as your brain's main fuel. There are two main types of diabetes: Type 1 and Type 2. Type 1 diabetes is an autoimmune condition where the body attacks insulin-producing cells in the pancreas, leading to little or no insulin production. Type 2 diabetes, which is more common, involves the body's inability to use insulin effectively, a condition known as insulin resistance. Over time, the pancreas can't make enough insulin to keep blood glucose at normal levels.

Several factors contribute to the development of diabetes, with lifestyle and genetic factors being the primary contributors. For Type 2 diabetes, being overweight or obese is a significant risk factor. Excess fat, especially when it's stored around the abdomen, can make cells more resistant to the effects of insulin. However, not everyone with Type 2 diabetes is overweight, and not everyone who is overweight will develop diabetes, indicating that genetics also play a role. Family history of diabetes can increase one's risk, suggesting a hereditary component to the disease.

Diet and physical activity are other crucial factors. Consuming a diet high in processed foods, sugar, and unhealthy fats can contribute to weight gain and increase the risk of developing insulin resistance. On the other hand, physical inactivity can exacerbate the situation by increasing obesity and insulin resistance. Regular physical activity helps control weight, uses up glucose as energy, and makes cells more sensitive to insulin.

For Type 1 diabetes, the exact cause is unknown, but it's believed to be a combination of genetic predisposition and environmental factors, such as viruses, that may trigger the immune system to attack the insulin-producing cells in the pancreas.

Another form of diabetes is gestational diabetes, which occurs during pregnancy. It's caused by hormonal changes during pregnancy along with genetic and lifestyle factors. Gestational diabetes can increase the risk of complications during pregnancy and delivery, but it usually resolves after giving birth. However, women who have had gestational diabetes have a higher risk of developing Type 2 diabetes later in life.

Prediabetes is a condition where blood sugar levels are higher than normal but not high enough to be classified as diabetes. Without intervention, prediabetes is likely to become Type 2 diabetes within a few years. Lifestyle changes, such as improving diet, increasing physical activity, and losing excess weight, can often reverse prediabetes and prevent the progression to Type 2 diabetes.

Understanding the causes and risk factors of diabetes is crucial for prevention and management. By adopting a healthier lifestyle, including a balanced diet, regular physical activity, and maintaining a healthy weight, individuals can significantly reduce their risk of developing Type 2 diabetes. For those already diagnosed, these lifestyle changes, along with medication if necessary, can help manage the condition and prevent complications.

Dr. Sebi's Approach to Treating Diabetes

Dr. Sebi's approach to treating diabetes centers on the body's inherent ability to heal itself when provided with the right natural resources. His methodology diverges from conventional treatments, focusing instead on a holistic, plant-based diet and specific herbs that target the root causes of diabetes, primarily insulin resistance and pancreatic health. By adhering to an alkaline diet, the body can achieve a state where it is better equipped to regulate blood sugar levels naturally. This diet eliminates harmful processed foods, sugars, and animal products that contribute to acidity and inflammation in the body, factors that are closely linked with the development and exacerbation of diabetes.

Key to this dietary shift is the inclusion of whole, nutrient-dense foods that are low on the glycemic index. These foods do not spike blood sugar levels rapidly and provide a sustained source of energy. Leafy greens, hemp seeds, walnuts, and burdock root are staples in this diet, rich in minerals and fiber that support blood sugar control and detoxification processes. Alkaline water and herbal teas are recommended to promote hydration and further aid in removing toxins from the body.

Dr. Sebi highlighted the importance of certain herbs in managing diabetes, such as Nopal (prickly pear cactus), which is known for its blood sugar-lowering properties, and cinnamon, which can improve insulin sensitivity. These herbs can be incorporated into the diet in various ways, including teas, capsules, and powders, making them a versatile addition to meals and beverages.

Physical activity, while not a direct part of Dr. Sebi's protocol, complements the dietary changes by improving insulin sensitivity and aiding in weight management. Engaging in regular, moderate exercise such as walking, yoga, or swimming can have profound effects on managing diabetes and enhancing overall health.

Dr. Sebi's approach also emphasizes the mental and emotional aspects of healing, advocating for stress reduction techniques and a positive outlook on life. Stress has a direct impact on blood sugar levels and managing stress through meditation, deep breathing exercises, and spending time in nature can help in maintaining a balanced state conducive to healing.

Transitioning to this lifestyle requires patience and dedication, with an understanding that the body needs time to adjust and heal. It is not a quick fix but a long-term commitment to living in a way that supports the body's natural healing processes. For those new to this way of living, it may be helpful to start slowly, incorporating one or two elements at a time and gradually building up to a full adoption of Dr. Sebi's recommendations.

While Dr. Sebi's approach has helped many in their journey towards health, it is crucial to consult with a healthcare provider before making significant changes, especially for those with existing health conditions or those taking medication for diabetes. This cannot be repeated enough. Monitoring blood sugar levels and adjusting the approach as needed also ensures safety and effectiveness in managing the condition.

By embracing Dr. Sebi's holistic approach to treating diabetes, individuals can empower themselves to take control of their health through natural, plant-based nutrition and lifestyle changes. This path not only addresses the symptoms of diabetes but also fosters an environment within the body that promotes overall well-being and vitality.

Specific Herbs and Foods for Diabetes Management

Managing diabetes naturally involves incorporating specific herbs and foods into your diet that can help regulate blood sugar levels and enhance insulin sensitivity. These natural remedies offer a holistic approach to diabetes management, aligning with Dr. Sebi's principles of using nature's bounty to support health and well-being. Here, we'll explore some of the most effective herbs and foods for diabetes management, providing practical ways to integrate them into your daily routine.

Bitter melon, with its distinct appearance and taste, stands out as a powerful food for managing diabetes. It contains three active substances with anti-diabetic properties that can help lower blood sugar levels. Incorporating bitter melon into your diet can be as simple as adding it to stir-fries or drinking it as a juice.

Cinnamon is another remarkable herb known for its ability to improve insulin sensitivity and lower blood sugar levels. Just a half teaspoon of cinnamon per day can have a positive effect. Sprinkle cinnamon on your morning oatmeal, add it to smoothies, or use it in baking to effortlessly reap its benefits.

Fenugreek seeds are highly valued for their fiber content, which can slow down the absorption of carbohydrates and sugars in the stomach, helping to regulate blood sugar levels. Soak fenugreek seeds overnight and consume them in the morning, or powder them and add to dishes for a subtle, beneficial spice.

Nopal or prickly pear cactus is another food recommended by Dr. Sebi for its blood sugar-lowering effects. It can be eaten grilled, boiled, or blended into smoothies. Its high fiber content helps with the slow release of sugar into the bloodstream.

Blueberries and other berries are rich in antioxidants and fiber, making them excellent for diabetes management. They can help improve insulin sensitivity and reduce the risk of developing diabetes. Enjoy them fresh as a snack, in smoothies, or mixed into a bowl of whole-grain cereal.

Avocado, with its healthy fats, can help improve insulin sensitivity. Incorporating avocado into your diet can be as simple as adding it to salads, spreading it on toast, or using it as a base for smoothies.

Lastly, green leafy vegetables like kale, lettuce (except for iceberg), and Swiss chard are nutrient-dense foods that are low in calories and carbohydrates, making them ideal for diabetes management. They can be easily added to smoothies, salads, or lightly sautéed as a side dish.

Incorporating these specific herbs and foods into your diet can significantly contribute to managing diabetes naturally. Remember, these dietary changes should complement your existing treatment plan. Always consult with a healthcare professional before making significant changes to your diet, especially if you are on medication for diabetes. By embracing these natural remedies, you can take an active role in managing your diabetes and improving your overall health.

4 Recipes for Healing Diabetes

5. Cinnamon and Clove Tea

Beneficial effects

Cinnamon and clove tea is a warming, aromatic beverage known for its potential to naturally manage blood sugar levels, making it an excellent choice for individuals looking to address diabetes. Cinnamon has been studied for its ability to improve insulin sensitivity and lower blood sugar levels, while cloves contain antioxidants that can aid in blood sugar control. Together, they create a powerful duo that not only tastes delightful but also supports metabolic health.

Portions	Preparation time	Cooking time
Makes about 2 servings	5 minutes	10 minutes

Ingredients

- 2 cinnamon sticks
- 1 teaspoon of whole cloves
- 4 cups of water

Instructions

1. In a medium-sized pot, bring 4 cups of water to a boil.
2. Once the water is boiling, add the cinnamon sticks and whole cloves.
3. Reduce the heat and let it simmer for about 10 minutes. This allows the flavors and beneficial compounds of the cinnamon and cloves to infuse into the water.
4. After simmering, remove the pot from the heat and strain the tea into cups or a teapot, discarding the cinnamon sticks and cloves.
5. Serve the tea warm and enjoy the soothing, aromatic flavors.

Variations

- For an extra flavor boost, add a slice of orange (common oranges only) or lemon to the tea while it simmers.

- Incorporate a slice of fresh ginger for additional digestive and anti-inflammatory benefits.

- If you prefer a stronger tea, allow the cinnamon and cloves to simmer for an additional 5 minutes before removing from heat.

Storage tips

If you have leftover tea, allow it to cool down before transferring it to a glass container. Store it in the refrigerator for up to 3 days. Reheat gently on the stove or enjoy chilled.

Tips for allergens

For those with allergies or sensitivities to cinnamon or cloves, herbal alternatives like rooibos tea can be used as a base for a similarly health-supportive beverage without these ingredients. Always consult with a healthcare provider before making significant changes to your diet, especially if managing a condition like diabetes.

Scientific references

- "Cinnamon: A Multifaceted Medicinal Plant," published in *Evidence-Based Complementary and Alternative Medicine*, highlights the potential of cinnamon in managing blood sugar levels and improving insulin sensitivity.

- "Antioxidant and Anti-inflammatory Properties of Capsaicin and Curcumin in Chronic Inflammation," found in the *Journal of Translational Medicine*, discusses the benefits of spices like cloves in managing inflammation, which is crucial for individuals with diabetes.

6. Fenugreek Seed Smoothie

Beneficial effects

This fenugreek seed smoothie is a nutritional powerhouse, especially beneficial for those managing diabetes. Fenugreek seeds are renowned for their natural ability to help lower blood sugar levels due to their high fiber content and other compounds that can improve insulin function. Incorporating this smoothie into your diet can aid in blood sugar management, while also providing a healthy dose of vitamins and minerals essential for overall health.

Portions	Preparation time
2 servings	10 minutes

Ingredients

- 2 tablespoons of fenugreek seeds, soaked overnight
- 1 cup of water
- 1 medium banana, ripe
- 1/2 cup of blueberries (fresh or frozen)
- 1 tablespoon of hemp seeds
- 1/2 teaspoon of cinnamon powder
- 1 teaspoon of agave syrup (optional, for sweetness)

Instructions

1. Begin by soaking the fenugreek seeds in water overnight. This softens the seeds and makes them easier to blend.
2. Drain the fenugreek seeds and add them to a blender.
3. Pour in the water.
4. Add the ripe banana, blueberries, hemp seeds, and cinnamon powder to the blender.
5. If you prefer a sweeter taste, add a teaspoon of agave syrup.
6. Blend on high speed until the mixture is smooth and creamy.
7. Taste the smoothie and adjust the sweetness if necessary by adding a little more agave syrup.
8. Serve immediately for the best flavor and nutrient retention.

Variations

- For an extra protein boost, add a scoop of your favorite plant-based protein powder.
- If you're not a fan of banana, you can substitute it with avocado for creaminess without the added sugar.

Storage tips

This smoothie is best enjoyed fresh. However, if you need to store it, keep it in an airtight container in the refrigerator for up to 24 hours. Give it a good stir or shake before drinking, as separation may occur.

Tips for allergens

- Ensure the agave syrup is pure and free from additives that might cause allergies.

Scientific references

- A study published in the *Journal of Medicinal Food* suggests that fenugreek seeds can significantly improve glucose tolerance and lower blood sugar levels due to their high soluble fiber content.

7. Bitter Melon Stir-Fry

Beneficial effects

Bitter melon stir-fry is a nutritious dish that harnesses the natural properties of bitter melon to help manage and treat diabetes. Bitter melon, known for its blood glucose-lowering effects, is an excellent addition to a diabetes management plan. This recipe combines bitter melon with other health-supportive ingredients to create a meal that not only helps regulate blood sugar levels, but also provides a rich source of dietary fiber, vitamins, and minerals essential for overall health.

Portions	Preparation time	Cooking time
Serves 2	10 minutes	15 minutes

Ingredients

- 1 medium bitter melon
- 2 tablespoons of olive oil
- 1/2 teaspoon of ground cumin
- 1 small onion, thinly sliced
- 1 red bell pepper, julienned
- 1 tablespoon of low-sodium soy sauce
- Salt to taste

Instructions

1. Cut the bitter melon in half lengthwise, scoop out the seeds with a spoon, and slice thinly.
2. Heat the olive oil in a large skillet over medium heat. Add the cumin, and sauté for about 1 minute until fragrant.
3. Add the sliced onion and red bell pepper to the skillet. Stir-fry for about 3-4 minutes until they start to soften.
4. Incorporate the sliced bitter melon into the skillet. Stir-fry for another 5-7 minutes until the bitter melon is tender but still crisp.
5. Drizzle the low-sodium soy sauce over the vegetables, and season with salt and pepper to taste. Stir well to ensure all the ingredients are evenly coated.
6. Remove from heat and transfer to a serving dish.

7. Serve warm as a side dish or over a bed of brown rice for a complete meal.

Variations

- Spice it up with a splash of chili sauce or a sprinkle of cayenne pepper flakes.
- Swap out the red bell pepper for other vegetables like snap peas for variety.

Storage tips

Store any leftovers in an airtight container in the refrigerator for up to 2 days. Reheat gently in a skillet or microwave before serving.

Tips for allergens

- For a gluten-free version, ensure the soy sauce is gluten-free or substitute with tamari.
- For those with soy allergies, use coconut aminos as a soy sauce alternative.

Scientific references

- A study published in the *Journal of Ethnopharmacology* found that consuming bitter melon can help reduce blood sugar levels in individuals with type 2 diabetes, highlighting its potential as a dietary supplement for diabetes management.

8. Coriander and Ginger Soup

Beneficial effects

This coriander and ginger soup harnesses the powerful anti-inflammatory and antioxidant properties of its key ingredient, ginger, to provide a healing and comforting remedy for those managing diabetes. Coriander may help lower blood sugar and cholesterol levels, supporting overall cardiovascular and digestive health. Ginger, on the other hand, has been shown to help reduce fasting blood sugar and improve hemoglobin A1c levels, making this soup an excellent dietary addition for diabetes management.

Portions	Preparation time	Cooking time
4 servings	15 minutes	25 minutes

Ingredients

- 2 tablespoons olive oil
- 1 large onion, finely chopped
- 1 tablespoon fresh ginger, grated
- 1 tablespoon coriander powder
- 1 teaspoon ground cumin
- 1 liter (about 4 cups) vegetable broth
- 1 cup carrots, chopped
- 1 cup sweet potatoes, cubed
- 1 can (15 oz) chickpeas, drained and rinsed
- Salt to taste

Instructions

1. Heat the olive oil in a large pot over medium heat. Add the onion and sautéing until the onion becomes translucent, about 5 minutes.
2. Stir in the grated ginger, coriander powder, and ground cumin, cooking for another 2 minutes until the spices are fragrant.
3. Pour in the vegetable broth and bring the mixture to a boil. Add the chopped carrots and cubed sweet potatoes to the pot.
4. Reduce the heat to a simmer and cook for about 15 minutes, or until the vegetables are tender.

5. Add the chickpeas to the pot and season with salt. Continue to simmer for another 5 minutes.
6. Once the vegetables are soft and the flavors have melded together, remove the pot from the heat.
7. Serve the soup in bowls.

Variations

- For a creamier texture, blend half of the soup before adding the chickpeas, then combine both parts.
- Add a squeeze of lemon juice before serving for a refreshing tang.
- For those who enjoy a bit of heat, include a pinch of cayenne pepper.

Storage tips

Store any leftover soup in an airtight container in the refrigerator for up to 3 days. Reheat on the stove or in the microwave when ready to eat.

Tips for allergens

- For those with allergies to chickpeas, lentils make a great substitute and offer similar nutritional benefits.
- Ensure the vegetable broth is gluten-free if necessary.

Scientific references

- "The Effect of Ginger on Fasting Blood Sugar, Hemoglobin A1c, Apolipoprotein B, Apolipoprotein A-I and Malondialdehyde in Type 2 Diabetic Patients," featured in the *Iranian Journal of Pharmaceutical Research*, highlights ginger's positive effects on blood sugar levels and diabetes management.

OVERCOMING LUPUS

Lupus, a complex and multifaceted disease, often leaves individuals feeling powerless due to its unpredictable nature. However, embracing Dr. Sebi's holistic approach can empower those affected to manage their symptoms and potentially reduce flare-ups. At the heart of this strategy lies the alkaline diet, complemented by specific herbs and lifestyle adjustments, all aimed at detoxifying the body and promoting an environment where healing can thrive.

The alkaline diet, rich in fruits, vegetables, nuts, and seeds, plays a pivotal role in managing lupus. This diet helps in reducing inflammation, a key factor in lupus flare-ups, by maintaining the body's pH at a slightly alkaline level. Foods like kale, wild rice, and walnuts are not only alkaline-forming but also packed with nutrients that support immune function and overall health. On the other hand, it's crucial to avoid acidic and inflammatory foods such as dairy, processed foods, and refined sugars, which can exacerbate symptoms.

Incorporating specific herbs into one's daily regimen is another cornerstone of Dr. Sebi's method. Herbs like burdock root, dandelion, and nettle possess powerful anti-inflammatory and detoxifying properties, making them invaluable in the fight against lupus. These herbs can be consumed as teas, tinctures, or supplements, offering a natural way to support the body's healing processes.

Detoxification is also a critical component of overcoming lupus. Regular detoxification aids in eliminating toxins from the body, thus reducing the burden on the immune system. Techniques such as fasting, consuming herbal teas, and engaging in gentle physical activities like yoga can facilitate this process. Additionally, ensuring adequate hydration by drinking plenty of spring water helps flush out toxins and supports cellular health.

Lifestyle adjustments are equally important in managing lupus. Stress, a known trigger for lupus flare-ups, can be mitigated through practices such as meditation, deep breathing exercises, and spending time in nature. Adequate sleep is also essential, as it allows the body to repair and regenerate. Creating a supportive community, whether through joining lupus support groups or connecting with others who follow Dr. Sebi's teachings, can provide emotional support and valuable insights.

By adopting Dr. Sebi's holistic approach, individuals with lupus can take proactive steps toward managing their condition. It's not merely about dietary changes but embracing a lifestyle that supports the body's natural healing capabilities. While lupus may not have a cure, following these principles can lead to significant improvements in quality of life, offering hope and empowerment to those affected. Remember, the journey to wellness is personal and requires patience, persistence, and a positive mindset.

What is Lupus and Its Symptoms

Lupus is an autoimmune disease where the body's immune system becomes hyperactive and attacks normal, healthy tissue. This results in symptoms such as inflammation, swelling, and damage to joints, skin, kidneys, blood, the heart, and lungs. In autoimmune diseases like lupus, the immune system mistakenly sees the body's own tissues as foreign invaders and decides to attack them. This leads to chronic (long-term) inflammation.

One of the hallmark symptoms of lupus is a facial rash that resembles the wings of a butterfly unfolding across both cheeks; however, not everyone with lupus will experience this symptom. Other common symptoms include extreme fatigue that doesn't go away with rest, headaches, swelling in the legs or around the eyes, pain in the chest when breathing deeply, and anemia (a condition where you have fewer red blood cells than normal). People with lupus may also experience sensitivity to the sun, with skin rashes or flare-ups after being in the sun.

Joint pain and stiffness are also prevalent in those with lupus, with swelling being a common complaint. The joints may feel stiff and uncomfortable, especially in the morning. Another significant aspect of lupus is its unpredictability; the symptoms can flare up, disappear, and then return. These flare-ups can be mild or severe, and they can make diagnosing lupus challenging.

Kidney involvement is among the more serious manifestations of lupus. The disease can affect the kidneys' ability to filter waste from the blood and can lead to conditions ranging from mild to life-threatening. The health of the kidneys in someone with lupus is closely monitored through urine and blood tests.

Neurological symptoms can also occur, including seizures, strokes, and episodes of psychosis. These symptoms, while less common, highlight the systemic nature of lupus, affecting not just one part of the body but multiple systems.

Lupus affects each individual differently. Some people may have only a few mild symptoms, and others may have many more severe symptoms. Symptoms can also be temporary or permanent. The most common strategy for managing lupus involves reducing inflammation through medication, lifestyle adjustments, and, in some cases, dietary changes to support overall health and reduce the likelihood of flare-ups.

Understanding lupus and its symptoms is the first step in managing this complex condition. Recognizing the signs early and consulting with a healthcare provider can lead to a diagnosis and a comprehensive treatment plan. Living with lupus requires adjustments, but with the right support and management strategies, individuals can lead active, fulfilling lives.

Dr. Sebi's Approach to Treating Lupus

Dr. Sebi's approach to treating lupus centers on the belief that a natural, alkaline-based diet, complemented by specific herbs and lifestyle adjustments, can significantly aid in managing the symptoms and potentially reducing the frequency of flare-ups. Recognizing lupus as an autoimmune condition where the body's immune system attacks its own tissues, Dr. Sebi's methodology focuses on reducing inflammation and detoxifying the body to promote healing and restore balance.

At the core of this approach is the adoption of an alkaline diet. This diet emphasizes the consumption of whole, plant-based foods that are rich in nutrients and naturally alkaline-forming. As has been mentioned previously, these include fruits, vegetables, nuts, and seeds, which work together to help maintain the body's pH at a slightly alkaline level. By doing so, this diet aims to reduce inflammation, a key contributor to lupus flare-ups, and support overall immune function. Foods particularly beneficial for individuals with lupus include leafy greens, such as kale, which is high in antioxidants and essential vitamins, and alkaline grains like quinoa and amaranth, which provide sustained energy and support gut health.

In addition to dietary changes, Dr. Sebi advocates for the use of specific herbs that have anti-inflammatory and detoxifying properties. Herbs such as burdock root, dandelion, and nettle are recommended for their ability to support kidney function, improve circulation, and aid in the removal of toxins from the body. These herbs can be consumed in various forms, including teas, tinctures, and capsules, offering a versatile and effective way to incorporate their healing properties into daily life.

Detoxification plays a crucial role in Dr. Sebi's approach to treating lupus. Regular detoxification helps in eliminating accumulated toxins from the body, thereby reducing the immune system's workload and potentially minimizing lupus symptoms. Techniques for detoxification include fasting, drinking herbal teas, and engaging in gentle physical activities such as yoga and walking. These practices not only aid in detoxification but also promote mental and emotional well-being, which is essential for managing a chronic condition like lupus.

Lifestyle adjustments are also a fundamental aspect of this holistic approach. Managing stress through meditation, deep breathing exercises, and spending time in nature can help mitigate one of the known triggers for lupus flare-ups. Ensuring adequate rest and sleep is vital for the body's healing and regeneration processes. Moreover, building a supportive community, whether through lupus support groups or networks of individuals following Dr. Sebi's teachings, can offer invaluable emotional support and encouragement.

By integrating these principles into daily life, individuals with lupus can take proactive steps toward managing their condition more effectively. It's important to remember that while this approach can lead to improvements in symptoms and overall well-being, it is not a cure for lupus. Patients are encouraged to work closely with their healthcare providers to monitor their condition and adjust their treatment plan as needed. Adopting Dr. Sebi's approach to treating lupus offers a complementary pathway to traditional medical treatments, emphasizing the power of natural healing and the importance of a holistic perspective on health.

Recommended Diet and Herbs

Adopting a diet that aligns with Dr. Sebi's principles involves focusing on whole, natural foods that support an alkaline environment within the body. This means prioritizing fresh fruits, vegetables, nuts, seeds, and grains that not only nourish the body, but also help maintain its natural balance. For individuals looking to embrace this lifestyle, incorporating specific foods and herbs into their daily routine can make a significant difference in their overall health and well-being.

Leafy greens such as kale and arugula are rich in minerals and essential vitamins, making them a cornerstone of the alkaline diet. These foods are not only alkaline-forming but also packed with antioxidants that support immune function and reduce inflammation. Alkaline grains like quinoa, amaranth, and wild rice offer a hearty base for meals while providing sustained energy and aiding in digestive health. Nuts and seeds, including walnuts and Brazil nuts, are excellent sources of healthy fats, protein, and fiber, contributing to a balanced diet.

Fruits play a crucial role in Dr. Sebi's recommended diet, with options like apples, berries, melons (seeded), and grapes offering a sweet treat that's also beneficial for the body. These fruits are high in vitamins, minerals, and hydration, making them perfect for snacking or adding to meals. It's important to consume a variety of fruits to take advantage of the wide range of nutrients they provide.

When it comes to herbs, Dr. Sebi highlighted several key options known for their healing properties. Burdock root, for instance, is celebrated for its blood-purifying and anti-inflammatory benefits. It can be consumed as a tea or added to meals for an extra nutrient boost. Dandelion, another powerful herb, supports liver function and aids in detoxification. Nettle is rich in vitamins and minerals, making it an excellent herb for supporting overall health and well-being. These herbs can be easily incorporated into daily routines, whether through teas, supplements, or as part of various dishes.

In addition to these specific foods and herbs, it's crucial to maintain hydration by drinking plenty of spring water throughout the day. Water not only supports detoxification but also ensures that the body's cells are properly nourished and functioning optimally.

Transitioning to an alkaline diet based on Dr. Sebi's recommendations may require some adjustments, but the benefits for health and well-being are well worth the effort. By focusing on whole, natural foods and incorporating specific herbs known for their healing properties, individuals can support their body's natural healing processes and promote a state of balance and health. Remember, the key to success with this diet is consistency and making choices that align with the body's needs. With patience and dedication, adopting an alkaline diet can be a transformative step toward improved health and vitality.

4 Recipes for Healing Lupus

9. Lupus Anti-Inflammatory Smoothie

Beneficial effects

This Lupus anti-inflammatory smoothie is crafted to help reduce inflammation associated with lupus, thanks to its blend of omega-3 fatty acids, antioxidants, and vitamins. The ingredients like mango, offer natural anti-inflammatory properties, while ginger adds digestive benefits and further inflammation relief. Incorporating this smoothie into your daily routine can aid in managing lupus symptoms, promoting overall well-being.

Portions	Preparation time
2 servings	10 minutes

Ingredients

- 1 cup mango, chopped
- 1/2 banana, ripe
- 1/2 inch piece of ginger, peeled
- 1 tablespoon flaxseed, ground
- 1 cup callaloo, fresh
- 1 cup coconut water

Instructions

1. Prepare the mango by chopping it into chunks.
2. Peel the banana and break it into pieces.
3. Peel the ginger and roughly chop it.
4. Place the mango, banana, ginger, ground flaxseed, and fresh callaloo into a blender.
5. Pour the coconut water over the ingredients in the blender.
6. Blend on high speed until the mixture becomes smooth and creamy.
7. If the smoothie is too thick, add more coconut water until you reach your desired consistency.

8. Taste and adjust the sweetness by adding a bit more banana if necessary.

9. Serve immediately for the best flavor and nutrient retention.

Variations

- For an extra protein boost, add a scoop of your favorite plant-based protein powder.

- If you prefer a colder smoothie, use frozen banana or add a few ice cubes before blending.

- Substitute kale for cucumber for a different nutrient profile.

Storage tips

This smoothie is best enjoyed fresh. However, if you need to store it, keep it in an airtight container in the refrigerator for up to 24 hours. Shake well before drinking, as separation may occur.

Tips for allergens

- For those with coconut allergies, substitute coconut water with almond milk or another non-dairy milk of your choice.

- Ensure the ground flaxseed is processed in a facility free from nuts, gluten, or other allergens that may affect you.

10. Elderberry and Chamomile Soothing Gel

Beneficial effects
This Elderberry and Chamomile Soothing Gel harnesses the powerful anti-inflammatory properties of chamomile along with the antioxidant benefits of elderberry. Perfect for those dealing with lupus, this gel can help reduce inflammation, soothe skin irritations, and promote healing of rashes or minor wounds often associated with lupus flare-ups. Chamomile is known for its soothing and skin-healing properties, while elderberry contributes to skin health with its high vitamin content and immune-boosting effects.

Preparation time
15 minutes

Ingredients
- 1/2 cup of elderberry syrup
- 1 teaspoon of chamomile extract
- 1 tablespoon of distilled water (optional, to adjust consistency)
- 10 drops of lavender essential oil (optional, for added soothing properties)

Instructions
- In a clean bowl, combine the elderberry syrup and chamomile extract. Mix thoroughly until well blended.
- If the mixture is too thick, slowly add distilled water, one teaspoon at a time, until you reach your desired consistency.
- If using, add the lavender essential oil to the mixture for its additional soothing and anti-inflammatory benefits. Stir well to combine.
- Transfer the gel to an airtight container.
- To use, apply a small amount of the gel to the affected area of the skin. Gently massage in a circular motion until absorbed.
- Use twice daily for best results, or as needed to soothe irritated skin

Variations
- For extra hydration, add a teaspoon of vitamin E oil to the mixture. Vitamin E can help nourish and protect the skin, enhancing the gel's healing properties.

- Incorporate raspberry extract for its antioxidant benefits and to enhance skin health further.

Storage tips

Store the Elderberry and Chamomile Soothing Gel in an airtight container in the refrigerator for up to 1 week. The cool temperature will also provide an additional soothing effect upon application.

Tips for allergens

- Always conduct a patch test before using the gel, especially if you have sensitive skin, to ensure there's no allergic reaction to the ingredients.

- Ensure that all extracts used are pure and free from contaminants that might cause skin irritation.

Scientific references

- Research has documented the benefits of elderberry and chamomile in various health publications, noting their roles in reducing inflammation and supporting skin health, particularly beneficial for conditions like lupus.

11. Omega-3 Rich Vegetable Stew

Beneficial effects

This Omega-3 Rich Vegetable Stew is designed to provide a hearty, nutritious meal that supports heart health and reduces inflammation, beneficial for individuals managing lupus. Omega-3 fatty acids, found abundantly in walnuts, hemp seeds, and flax seeds, are known for their anti-inflammatory properties and ability to improve cardiovascular health. This stew combines the goodness of these omega-3-rich seeds and nuts with a variety of vegetables, making it a balanced meal that promotes overall well-being.

Portions	Preparation time	Cooking time
4 servings	15 minutes	30 minutes

Ingredients

- 2 tablespoons olive oil
- 1 large onion, chopped
- 1 red bell pepper, diced
- 2 carrots, sliced
- 2 potatoes, cubed
- 1 teaspoon dried thyme
- 1 teaspoon dried oregano
- 1 bay leaf
- 4 cups vegetable broth
- 1 cup diced tomatoes (canned or fresh)
- 1/2 cup walnuts, chopped
- 1/4 cup hemp seeds
- 1 tablespoon flax seeds, ground
- Salt to taste
- Fresh dill, chopped (for garnish)

Instructions

1. Heat the olive oil in a large pot over medium heat. Add the onion and sauté until the onion is translucent, about 5 minutes.

2. Add the red bell pepper, carrots, and potatoes to the pot. Cook for another 5 minutes, stirring occasionally.
3. Stir in the thyme, oregano, and bay leaf. Pour in the vegetable broth and bring the mixture to a boil.
4. Reduce the heat to a simmer and add the diced tomatoes, walnuts, hemp seeds, and ground flax seeds. Season with salt.
5. Cover and simmer for about 20 minutes, or until the vegetables are tender.
6. Remove the bay leaf and discard. Taste the stew and adjust the seasoning if necessary.
7. Serve hot, garnished with fresh dill.

Variations

- For added greens, include a handful of chopped kale or spinach during the last 5 minutes of cooking.

- Include a splash of lemon juice for added brightness and a vitamin C boost.

- For a spicier stew, add a pinch of cayenne pepper or a few slices of jalapeño.

Storage tips

Store any leftovers in an airtight container in the refrigerator for up to 3 days. Reheat gently on the stove or in the microwave, adding a little extra broth or water if the stew has thickened too much.

Tips for allergens

- Ensure all ingredients used are free from contaminants and suitable for those with specific dietary restrictions, such as gluten-free or nut-free requirements.

Scientific references

- Studies in the *Journal of the American College of Nutrition* have shown that omega-3 fatty acids can significantly reduce inflammation and may help manage symptoms associated with autoimmune diseases like lupus.

- Research in the *European Journal of Clinical Nutrition* highlights the role of omega-3 fatty acids in cardiovascular health, suggesting benefits for those with lupus, who may be at increased risk for heart disease.

12. Ginger and Fennel Tea

Beneficial effects

Ginger and Fennel Tea is a soothing and anti-inflammatory beverage that leverages the powerful properties of its main ingredients to support overall health. Fennel, known for its digestive benefits and anti-inflammatory properties, pairs well with ginger, which improves digestion and reduces nausea. Together, they create a tea that not only warms the soul but also supports the body's immune system and reduces inflammation, making it particularly beneficial for those managing conditions like lupus.

Portions	Preparation time	Cooking time
2 servings	5 minutes	10 minutes

Ingredients

- 1 tablespoon fennel seeds
- 1 inch fresh ginger root, thinly sliced or grated
- 4 cups of water
- Lemon slice for garnish (optional)

Instructions

1. Bring the water to a boil in a medium-sized saucepan.
2. Add the sliced or grated ginger and fennel seeds to the boiling water.
3. Reduce the heat and simmer for about 10 minutes to allow the flavors and beneficial compounds to infuse into the water.
4. Strain the tea into mugs, discarding the solids.
5. Garnish with a slice of lemon for an extra boost of vitamin C and flavor.
6. Enjoy the tea warm, ideally in the morning or before bedtime.

Variations

- Add a cinnamon stick during the simmering process for a warming, spicy flavor that also offers additional blood sugar regulation benefits.
- For those who prefer a creamier tea, add a splash of coconut milk before serving for a rich, smooth texture and a hint of sweetness.

Storage tips

This tea is best enjoyed fresh, but you can store any leftovers in the refrigerator for up to 2 days. Reheat gently on the stove or enjoy cold as a refreshing cayenne pepper and ginger tonic.

Tips for allergens

For those with allergies or sensitivities, this tea is naturally free from common allergens such as dairy, gluten, and nuts. However, always ensure that any added sweeteners or garnishes meet your dietary needs.

Scientific references

- "Ginger on Human Health: A Comprehensive Systematic Review of 109 Randomized Controlled Trials," found in *Nutrients*, discusses the various health benefits of ginger, including its anti-inflammatory properties.

- Research highlights the benefits of fennel in aiding digestion and its anti-inflammatory effects, supporting its use in herbal remedies and dietary supplements.

LOWERING HIGH BLOOD PRESSURE

High blood pressure, also known as hypertension, is a common condition where the force of the blood against your artery walls is high enough that it may eventually cause health problems, such as heart disease. It's often referred to as the "silent killer" because it typically has no symptoms but can lead to serious health issues. Dr. Sebi's approach to lowering high blood pressure focuses on natural, holistic methods, emphasizing the importance of diet, lifestyle changes, and the use of specific herbs to manage and potentially reduce high blood pressure.

The foundation of Dr. Sebi's method for combating high blood pressure lies in the adoption of an alkaline diet. This diet encourages the consumption of whole, plant-based foods that help to maintain the body's natural alkaline balance. Foods that are particularly beneficial for those with high blood pressure include leafy greens, such as kale, which is high in magnesium, a mineral that can help to relax blood vessel walls and reduce blood pressure. Other alkaline-forming foods recommended are beets, bananas, and berries, all known for their blood pressure-lowering effects. These foods are rich in potassium, which helps to balance out the negative effects of salt in the diet and ease tension in the blood vessels.

In addition to dietary changes, Dr. Sebi advocated for the reduction of salt intake. Excessive salt consumption can cause the body to retain water, which in turn increases blood pressure. By limiting salt and replacing it with herbs and spices to flavor food, individuals can significantly reduce their blood pressure levels. It's also important to eliminate processed and fried foods from the diet, as these are typically high in unhealthy fats and sodium, which can exacerbate high blood pressure.

Dr. Sebi also highlighted the importance of hydration. Drinking plenty of spring water throughout the day helps to flush toxins from the body and maintain a healthy blood volume, contributing to lower blood pressure levels. Hydration is key to ensuring that the body's systems are functioning optimally and can effectively manage blood pressure.

Lifestyle adjustments play a crucial role in managing high blood pressure. Regular physical activity, such as walking, yoga, or swimming, can help to lower blood pressure by strengthening the heart, enabling it to pump blood more efficiently. Stress management techniques, including meditation and deep breathing exercises, are also beneficial. Stress can cause temporary spikes in blood pressure, so finding ways to relax and manage stress is essential for long-term blood pressure control.

Dr. Sebi recommended several herbs known for their blood pressure-lowering properties. These include hawthorn berry, which has been shown to improve cardiovascular health, and others like basil, cinnamon, and cardamom.

By integrating these principles into daily life, individuals can take significant steps toward lowering their high blood pressure naturally. It's important to remember that while these methods can be effective, they should complement and not replace any treatment plans prescribed by a healthcare provider. Regular monitoring of blood pressure and consultation with a healthcare professional are crucial to safely managing high blood pressure.

Adopting Dr. Sebi's holistic approach to health can empower individuals to take control of their blood pressure and overall well-being. Through a combination of dietary changes, lifestyle adjustments, and the use of specific herbs, it's possible to reduce high blood pressure and reduce the risk of heart disease and other related health issues. This natural, holistic path offers a promising alternative for those seeking to manage their high blood pressure without relying solely on medication.

Causes and Symptoms of High Blood Pressure

High blood pressure, also known as hypertension, occurs when the force of your blood pushing against the walls of your blood vessels is consistently too high. This condition can lead to a host of health issues, including heart disease, stroke, and kidney failure, making it imperative to understand its causes and symptoms for effective management and prevention.

One of the primary causes of high blood pressure is an unhealthy diet, particularly one high in salt, processed foods, and fatty foods. These dietary choices can increase the volume of blood or the amount of resistance in your blood vessels, leading to higher blood pressure. Additionally, a lack of physical activity can contribute to hypertension by making the heart work harder to pump blood through the body, which can stiffen or narrow the blood vessels over time.

Obesity is another significant factor, as it requires more blood to supply oxygen and nutrients to the body, increasing the volume of blood flowing through your blood vessels. This additional strain can raise blood pressure. Moreover, excessive alcohol consumption and tobacco use can damage the heart and blood vessels, leading to increased blood pressure. Certain medical conditions, such as diabetes and kidney disease, can also contribute to hypertension by affecting how your body manages fluids and salts or by causing damage to your blood vessels.

Genetics and family history play a role as well, with hypertension running in families, suggesting a genetic component to the condition. Age is another factor, with the risk of high blood pressure increasing as you get older due to the natural hardening and narrowing of the arteries.

Stress can temporarily increase blood pressure by causing the heart to beat faster and narrowing the blood vessels. Though the long-term effects of stress on blood pressure are not fully understood, it is believed that managing stress can help control blood pressure.

Symptoms of high blood pressure are often silent, earning it the nickname "the silent killer." Many people with hypertension may not experience any symptoms and may only discover their condition during a routine health checkup. However, some individuals with high blood pressure may experience headaches, shortness of breath, nosebleeds, or flushing. These symptoms typically do not occur until high blood pressure has reached a severe or life-threatening stage.

Understanding the causes and recognizing the potential lack of symptoms associated with high blood pressure underscores the importance of regular blood pressure screenings. Early detection and management through lifestyle changes, such as adopting a healthier diet, increasing physical activity, and reducing salt intake, can significantly reduce the risk of developing the severe health complications associated with hypertension.

Dietary and Lifestyle Recommendations

Adopting a heart-healthy diet and making positive lifestyle changes are foundational steps in managing high blood pressure. Emphasizing the consumption of whole, plant-based foods while reducing intake of salt, proces-

Embracing natural herbs and remedies is not just about treating specific health issues, but also about nurturing your body and mind, promoting a state of balance and harmony. As you begin to explore the world of natural healing, you'll discover the profound impact these simple yet powerful plants can have on your health journey, offering a path toward a more vibrant, healthy life.

4 Recipes to Reduce High Blood Pressure

13. Dandelion Greens and Thyme Infusion

Beneficial effects

This potent natural remedy uses dandelion greens and thyme to support cardiovascular health. Dandelion greens are known for their diuretic properties, helping the body eliminate excess fluid and reducing strain on the heart. Thyme complements this by offering antioxidants that can improve heart health and potentially lower blood pressure levels. Together, they form a powerful duo that promotes a healthy cardiovascular system and maintains blood pressure levels.

Portions	Preparation time	Cooking time
2 servings	5 minutes	10 minutes

Ingredients

- 4 cups of water
- 1/4 cup of fresh dandelion greens, chopped
- 1 tablespoon of fresh thyme leaves

Instructions

1. Bring the water to a boil in a medium-sized pot.
2. Add the chopped dandelion greens and thyme leaves to the boiling water and reduce the heat. Let it simmer for about 10 minutes.
3. Remove the pot from the heat and strain the infusion into cups, discarding the solids.
4. Enjoy the infusion warm, ideally in the morning or before bedtime.

Variations

- For an added flavor and health boost, include a slice of key lime or a dash of cayenne pepper to the infusion.

- For a deeper flavor, steep the infusion with a bay leaf, removing it before drinking.

Storage tips

This infusion is best enjoyed fresh, but if you need to store it, keep it in an airtight container in the refrigerator for up to 24 hours. Reheat gently on the stove or enjoy chilled.

Tips for allergens

- For those sensitive to certain sweeteners, enjoy the infusion without any additives to maintain its natural benefits.

Scientific references

- Research in various journals suggests that dandelion greens have a diuretic effect which can be beneficial in managing hypertension by reducing blood volume and pressure.

- Studies have also shown that thyme contains compounds that may help reduce blood pressure and improve overall heart health.

14. Hibiscus and Lemon Tea

Beneficial effects

Hibiscus and lemon tea is a refreshing beverage known for its potential to lower high blood pressure naturally. Hibiscus contains bioactive compounds that have been shown to reduce blood pressure by acting as natural ACE inhibitors, similar to some medications used for treating hypertension. Lemon adds a vitamin C boost, which is associated with **beneficial effects** on heart health and blood pressure regulation. Together, they create a delicious tea that not only hydrates but also supports cardiovascular health.

Portions	Preparation time	Cooking time
2 servings	5 minutes	10 minutes

Ingredients

- 4 cups of water
- 2 tablespoons of dried hibiscus flowers
- 1 tablespoon of fresh lemon juice

Instructions

1. Bring the water to a boil in a medium-sized pot.
2. Once boiling, add the dried hibiscus flowers to the pot.
3. Reduce the heat and let it simmer for about 10 minutes.
4. Remove from heat and strain the tea into a pitcher or directly into serving cups, discarding the hibiscus flowers.
5. Stir in the fresh lemon juice.
6. Serve the tea warm, or chill it in the refrigerator for a refreshing cold drink.

Variations

- For a spicy twist, add a cinnamon stick or a few slices of fresh ginger to the pot while simmering the hibiscus flowers.
- Mix in a splash of orange juice for a fruity variation.

Storage tips

If you have leftover tea, store it in a sealed container in the refrigerator for up to 5 days. Enjoy it cold, or reheat gently on the stove or in the microwave.

Tips for allergens

This recipe is naturally free from common allergens, including dairy, gluten, nuts, and soy.

Scientific references

- A study published in the *Journal of Nutrition* found that consuming hibiscus tea lowered blood pressure in a group of prehypertensive and mildly hypertensive adults.

- Research in the *American Journal of Clinical Nutrition* highlights the role of vitamin C, found in lemon, in reducing blood pressure and promoting arterial health.

15. Beetroot and Ginger Juice

Beneficial effects

Beetroot and ginger juice is a potent combination aimed at reducing high blood pressure naturally. Beetroot is rich in nitrates that help relax blood vessels and improve blood flow, while ginger is known for its anti-inflammatory and blood-pressure-lowering effects. Together, they create a powerful drink that can help manage hypertension and support cardiovascular health.

Portions	Preparation time
2 servings	10 minutes

Ingredients

- 2 medium beetroots, peeled and chopped
- 1 inch piece of ginger, peeled
- 1 apple, cored and sliced (for sweetness)
- 1/2 lemon, juiced
- 1 cup of water or coconut water (for blending)

Instructions

1. Place the chopped beetroots, peeled ginger, sliced apple (but not Granny Smith or Red Delicious), and lemon juice into a blender.
2. Add 1 cup of water or coconut water to help the ingredients blend smoothly.
3. Blend on high until the mixture is completely smooth.
4. Use a fine mesh strainer or cheesecloth to strain the juice into a large bowl, pressing down to extract as much liquid as possible.
5. Discard the pulp or save it for use in compost or baking.
6. Pour the juice into glasses and serve immediately for the freshest taste and maximum health benefits.

Variations

- Add a handful of kale for an extra nutrient boost without significantly altering the taste.
- For a sweeter juice, include an extra apple or a small amount of pure agave syrup.

- A pinch of cayenne pepper can be added for those who prefer a spicy kick, which also boosts metabolism.

Storage tips

This juice is best enjoyed fresh but can be stored in an airtight container in the refrigerator for up to 24 hours. Shake well before serving if separation occurs.

Tips for allergens

- For those with allergies to citrus, omit the lemon juice or substitute it with a small amount of apple cider vinegar for a similar zesty flavor.

- Ensure the use of fresh, organic ingredients to minimize exposure to pesticides and other chemicals.

Scientific references

- A study published in the *Journal of Nutrition* found that beetroot juice lowers blood pressure in individuals with hypertension, attributing the effect to its high nitrate content.

- Research in the *International Journal of Cardiology* has shown ginger's effectiveness in lowering blood pressure and its potential role in cardiovascular health protection.

16. Celery and Cucumber Smoothie

Beneficial effects

The celery and cucumber Smoothie is a refreshing and hydrating drink, perfect for lowering high blood pressure. Celery contains phthalides, which can help relax the muscles around arteries and allow those vessels to dilate, providing more space for the blood to flow, thus reducing pressure. Cucumbers are high in potassium, which can help lower blood pressure by balancing out the negative effects of sodium. This smoothie is an excellent way to incorporate these health benefits into your diet in a delicious and convenient way.

Portions	Preparation time
2 servings	10 minutes

Ingredients

- 2 cups chopped celery
- 1 large cucumber, peeled and chopped
- 1/2 green apple, cored and chopped
- 1 tablespoon fresh lemon juice
- 1/2 cup of water or coconut water
- A handful of fresh parsley
- Ice cubes (optional)

Instructions

1. Place the chopped celery, cucumber, and green apple into a blender.
2. Add the fresh lemon juice and water or coconut water to the blender.
3. Add a handful of fresh parsley for an extra health boost.
4. Blend on high speed until the mixture becomes smooth and creamy.
5. If you prefer a colder smoothie, add a few ice cubes and blend again until smooth.
6. Taste the smoothie, and if needed, adjust the sweetness by adding a bit more apple.
7. Serve immediately for the best flavor and nutrient retention.

Variations

- For an extra kick, add a small piece of ginger or a pinch of cayenne pepper before blending.

- Include a scoop of protein powder to make this smoothie a more filling breakfast or snack option.

- Swap out the green apple for a pear for a different flavor profile.

Storage tips

It's best to consume the smoothie immediately after blending to ensure maximum freshness and nutrient intake. However, if you need to store it, keep it in an airtight container in the refrigerator for up to 24 hours. Shake well before drinking, as separation may occur.

Tips for allergens

- For those with allergies to celery, substitute with more cucumber for a green nutrient boost.

- Ensure the protein powder (if used) is free from allergens that may affect you, such as gluten, dairy, or soy.

COMBATING CANCER WITH NATURAL METHODS

Cancer, a word that strikes fear into the hearts of many, is often seen as an insurmountable enemy. However, adopting natural methods to combat this disease can empower individuals, offering hope and a sense of control over their health. Dr. Sebi's holistic approach to cancer focuses on creating an internal environment where cancer cells cannot thrive. This involves a combination of dietary changes, herbal remedies, and lifestyle adjustments aimed at detoxifying the body and enhancing its natural healing capabilities.

At the forefront of this approach is the alkaline diet, which emphasizes the consumption of electric foods—those that are natural, unprocessed, and rich in vitamins, minerals, and antioxidants. These foods help to maintain the body's pH at an alkaline level, which is inhospitable to cancer cells. Key components of this diet include leafy greens, fruits, nuts, seeds, and whole grains. These foods not only support the body's alkaline state but also provide the nutrients needed for optimal health and immune function.

Herbs play a crucial role in Dr. Sebi's cancer-fighting regimen. Soursop leaf, burdock root, and dandelion are just a few examples of herbs known for their anti-cancer properties. Soursop leaf, in particular, has been studied for its ability to target and kill cancer cells without harming healthy cells. These herbs can be consumed in various forms, such as teas, tinctures, or capsules, making them a versatile addition to any cancer prevention or treatment plan.

Detoxification is another pillar of combating cancer naturally. Regular detox helps to eliminate toxins and waste products from the body, reducing the load on the immune system and allowing it to focus on healing. Techniques such as fasting, consuming herbal teas, and engaging in gentle exercises like yoga and walking are effective ways to support the body's detoxification processes. Additionally, ensuring adequate hydration by drinking plenty of spring water is essential for flushing out toxins and supporting overall cellular health.

Lifestyle adjustments are equally important in the fight against cancer. Stress, for example, can weaken the immune system and create an environment conducive to cancer growth. Incorporating stress-reduction techniques such as meditation, deep breathing exercises, and spending time in nature can help to lower stress levels and improve the body's ability to fight cancer. Adequate sleep is also crucial, as it allows the body to repair and regenerate. Creating a supportive community, whether through joining cancer support groups or connecting with others who are following a similar healing journey, can provide emotional support and valuable insights.

By embracing Dr. Sebi's holistic approach to health, individuals can take proactive steps toward preventing and combating cancer. It's important to remember that this approach is not a substitute for conventional cancer treatments, but rather a complementary pathway that emphasizes the power of natural healing. Working closely with healthcare providers to monitor the condition and adjust treatment plans as needed is crucial. With patience, dedication, and a positive mindset, adopting a natural, holistic approach to cancer can lead to improvements in health and well-being, offering hope and empowerment to those affected by this disease.

Understanding Cancer from a Holistic Perspective

Cancer from a holistic perspective is viewed not just as a collection of symptoms or a specific diagnosis but as a signal from the body that there is an imbalance that needs to be addressed. This approach considers the entire person, their body, mind, and spirit, and seeks to restore harmony and health through natural and non-invasive methods. The holistic view suggests that cancer, like many other diseases, arises from an environment within the body that has become conducive to disease due to a variety of factors including diet, lifestyle, stress, and exposure to toxins.

A key principle in this perspective is the belief that the body has an inherent ability to heal itself when given the right conditions. Creating an internal environment that is hostile to cancer involves several strategies that work together to boost the body's natural defenses and repair mechanisms. This includes nourishing the body with alkaline foods that are rich in nutrients, minimizing exposure to toxins, managing stress, and fostering positive emotional and mental health.

The diet plays a crucial role in creating an alkaline environment that is less favorable for cancer cells to thrive. Foods that are highly processed, high in sugar, or contain artificial additives contribute to acidity and inflammation, which can support the growth of cancer cells. On the other hand, a diet rich in organic fruits, vegetables, whole grains, and seeds provides essential nutrients and antioxidants that support cellular health and reduce inflammation.

Detoxification is another important aspect of the holistic approach to cancer. Regularly cleansing the body of toxins through specific detox diets, herbal teas, and fasting can help to reduce the toxic load on the body and support the immune system. Physical activities and exercises that increase blood flow and lymphatic drainage also play a role in detoxification, helping to remove waste products and improve oxygenation to tissues.

Stress management is equally important, as chronic stress can weaken the immune system and create an environment that is more susceptible to cancer. Techniques such as meditation, yoga, deep breathing exercises, and spending time in nature can help to reduce stress and promote a sense of well-being. Adequate sleep and rest are also vital for allowing the body to repair and regenerate.

Creating a supportive community and fostering positive relationships can provide emotional support and reduce feelings of isolation and stress that often accompany a cancer diagnosis. Engaging in activities that bring joy and fulfillment, pursuing creative outlets, and connecting with others who share similar values and lifestyles can contribute to a positive outlook and enhance the healing process.

In embracing a holistic approach to cancer, it is important to work closely with healthcare professionals who are supportive of integrating natural and conventional treatments. This ensures that all aspects of health are considered and that any treatments or interventions are safe and complementary. With patience and commitment, adopting a holistic approach to health can lead to significant improvements in well-being and quality of life, offering hope and empowerment to those facing cancer.

Dr. Sebi's Cancer Treatment Protocols

Dr. Sebi's cancer treatment protocols are grounded in the principle that a holistic approach, focusing on natural and alkaline-rich foods, can significantly alter the body's internal environment, making it less conducive for cancer cells to grow and proliferate. Central to this protocol is the emphasis on an alkaline diet, which involves consuming foods that not only nourish the body but also maintain its pH at a level where cancer cells find it difficult to survive. This diet is rich in leafy greens, fruits, nuts, seeds, and whole grains, all of which are integral to creating an alkaline state within the body.

Incorporating specific herbs with anti-cancer properties is another cornerstone of Dr. Sebi's approach. Herbs such as soursop leaf, burdock root, and dandelion are celebrated for their ability to target and neutralize cancer cells. These herbs, available in various forms like teas, tinctures, and capsules, are chosen for their potent antioxidant properties, which play a crucial role in detoxifying the body and bolstering the immune system against cancer.

Detoxification is a process that Dr. Sebi strongly advocates for, emphasizing its importance in cleansing the body of toxins and waste products that can burden the immune system. Regular detox through fasting, herbal teas, and the consumption of alkaline water aids in reducing the body's toxic load, thereby enhancing its natural healing capabilities. Engaging in physical activities that promote detoxification, such as yoga and walking, further supports the body's efforts to cleanse itself.

Lifestyle modifications form an integral part of Dr. Sebi's cancer treatment protocols. Stress management techniques, including meditation and deep breathing exercises, are encouraged to mitigate the adverse effects of stress on the body's immune function. Adequate rest and sleep are also highlighted for their roles in allowing the body to repair and regenerate, crucial processes in the fight against cancer. Building a supportive community, whether through cancer support groups or connections with others embracing a similar health journey, provides emotional support that is vital for healing.

By adhering to these protocols, individuals are empowered to take proactive steps towards preventing and combating cancer through natural means. It is essential, however, to approach this journey with patience and to maintain open communication with healthcare providers to ensure that the natural regimen complements any existing treatments. Dr. Sebi's protocols are not intended to replace conventional cancer treatments but to offer a complementary pathway that harnesses the power of natural healing. Through dedication to these principles, individuals can enhance their body's resilience, improve their overall well-being, and embark on a hopeful path towards recovery and health.

Detoxifying the Body to Prevent Cancer

Detoxifying the body plays a pivotal role in creating an environment where cancer is less likely to thrive. This process involves eliminating toxins and waste products that accumulate over time due to factors such as diet, lifestyle, and exposure to environmental pollutants. By focusing on detoxification, we support our body's natural ability to cleanse itself, which is crucial for maintaining optimal health and preventing diseases, including cancer.

The first step in detoxifying the body is to reduce the intake of substances that contribute to the toxic load. This means opting for organic foods whenever possible to avoid pesticides and chemicals found in conventional produce. It also involves minimizing processed foods, which are often high in sugar, unhealthy fats, and additives, all of which can contribute to inflammation and an acidic environment conducive to cancer growth. Instead, prioritize whole, nutrient-dense foods that nourish the body and support detoxification processes.

Hydration is another key component of detoxification. Drinking adequate amounts of clean, filtered water helps to flush toxins from the body through the kidneys and supports all bodily functions. Incorporating herbal teas such as dandelion or green tea can also aid in detoxification, thanks to their diuretic properties and high antioxidant content.

Regular physical activity is essential for promoting detoxification. Exercise increases blood circulation and encourages sweating, another effective way to eliminate toxins. Activities like yoga and rebounding are particularly beneficial as they also support lymphatic drainage, helping the body to rid itself of waste products more efficiently.

Fasting or following a detoxification diet for a short period can further aid in cleansing the body. These practices give the digestive system a break, allowing the body to focus its energy on healing and detoxification. During a detox diet, consuming alkaline foods, fresh juices, and smoothies can provide essential nutrients while supporting the body's natural detox pathways.

Herbal supplements and teas can be powerful allies in the detoxification process. Herbs such as milk thistle and burdock root have been shown to support liver function, a key organ in the body's detoxification system. These herbs can be taken in supplement form or used to make healing teas.

It's also important to consider the role of mental and emotional health in the detoxification process. Stress can negatively impact the body's ability to detoxify by hindering digestive and immune functions. Incorporating stress-reduction techniques such as meditation, deep breathing exercises, and spending time in nature can help to reduce the overall toxic burden on the body.

Creating a supportive environment is crucial for successful detoxification. This includes not only the physical environment, such as ensuring clean air and water, but also a supportive social environment. Connecting with a community of like-minded individuals can provide encouragement and motivation to maintain a detoxifying lifestyle.

By adopting these practices, individuals can significantly enhance their body's natural detoxification processes, creating an internal environment that is less hospitable to cancer cells. While detoxification is not a cure-all, it is a powerful tool in the prevention and holistic management of cancer, empowering individuals to take an active role in their health and well-being. Remember, these strategies should complement, not replace, the guidance and treatment plans provided by healthcare professionals.

Nutritional Recommendations for Cancer Patients

For cancer patients, nutrition plays a pivotal role in supporting the body through the challenges of treatment and recovery. Emphasizing a diet rich in alkaline foods can help create an environment less conducive to cancer growth while providing the necessary nutrients to bolster the immune system and enhance overall well-being. Key to this approach is focusing on whole, unprocessed foods that are dense in nutrients and possess natural anti-inflammatory and antioxidant properties.

Leafy greens such as kale and collard greens are foundational to an alkaline diet, offering high levels of vitamins, minerals, and fiber with minimal calories. These greens support detoxification processes in the liver and contribute to an alkaline environment in the body. Including a variety of colors in your diet through vegetables like beets, and sweet potatoes ensures a broad spectrum of phytonutrients, essential for combating oxidative stress and reducing inflammation.

Fruits, while slightly more acidic, are still an important part of a cancer-fighting diet. Berries, in particular, are packed with antioxidants and vitamins that support immune health and can protect cells from damage. Avocados, rich in healthy fats and low in sugar, provide essential fatty acids that support cell membrane health and can help in the absorption of fat-soluble vitamins.

Nuts and seeds are another crucial component, offering protein, healthy fats, and vital minerals. For example, walnuts not only provide protein and healthy fats but also contain fiber, which aids in digestion and helps maintain a healthy gut microbiome, crucial for immune function and detoxification.

Whole grains, such as quinoa, millet, and amaranth, are preferred over refined grains because they maintain their nutrient content and provide the body with steady energy. These grains are also rich in fiber, supporting digestive health and helping to regulate blood sugar levels, which is particularly important for cancer patients who may experience fluctuations in energy.

Hydration is another key aspect of nutrition for cancer patients. Drinking plenty of alkaline water or herbal teas can help flush toxins from the body and support cellular hydration. Lemon water, despite its initial acidity, becomes alkaline in the body and can help to maintain the body's pH balance.

Incorporating specific herbs and spices into the diet can further support the body's fight against cancer. Ginger, another powerful anti-inflammatory, can help alleviate nausea, a common side effect of cancer treatments. Other herbs like dandelion greens can support liver function and detoxification.

For cancer patients, it's also important to listen to the body and adjust dietary choices to meet changing needs and preferences. Treatment side effects may alter taste preferences or affect appetite, making it necessary to find palatable ways to incorporate these nutritious foods. Working with a nutritionist or dietitian who is familiar with cancer care can provide personalized guidance and ensure that dietary choices support healing and recovery.

Embracing a diet centered around whole, alkaline foods can empower cancer patients, providing the nutrients needed for strength and resilience during treatment and beyond. While nutrition is just one aspect of a comprehensive approach to cancer care, it offers a powerful tool for supporting the body's natural healing processes and improving quality of life.

Thank You For Your Support!

★★★★★

I'm eager to know what you think!

Simply **scan this QR code** to jump straight to my book's review page on Amazon.

Your insights are invaluable – they aid in my growth as an author and assist others in discovering this book.

Feel free to **share a photo or video review showcasing you with the book**. Your experience could inspire others to embark on their adventure with my book!

Rosalinda

BONUS EXTRA!!!

Scan the QR CODE

and Get Your **Dr. Sebi's Alkaline and Anti-Inflammatory Diet Transformation for Beginners E-book** and **Dr. Sebi's 7-Day Full-Body Detox Plan** -
All Straight into Your Email!!

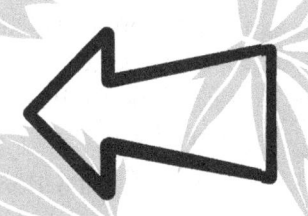

As SPAM Filters Are Pretty Crazy These Days...
...WHITELIST this Email Address!

info@greenessencepublishing.com

In This Way, Your Bonus Will Appear in the Main Folder of Your INBOX and They Will Not Be Buried Along With Other Advertisements in Your PROMOTION/SPAM Folder.

HERE IS HOW TO DO IT:
From Android Smartphone/Tablet
Open the Contacts App;
In the lower right corner, tap + (Add);
Enter the name and email address and then tap Save.

From iPhone/iPad
Open the Contacts App;
In the upper right corner, tap + (Add);
Enter the name and email address and then tap Finish.

4 Recipes for Healing Cancer

17. Anti-Cancer Green Juice

Beneficial effects

The anti-cancer green juice is a powerful blend designed to support the body's natural defenses against cancer. Rich in antioxidants, vitamins, and minerals, this juice can help neutralize harmful free radicals and reduce inflammation, which are key factors in cancer prevention and support during cancer treatment. Ingredients like kale offer high levels of vitamin C and beta-carotene, while ginger and lemon add detoxifying and immune-boosting properties.

Portions	Preparation time
2 servings	10 minutes

Ingredients

- 1 cup of kale, chopped
- 1 green apple, cored and sliced
- 1/2 cucumber, chopped
- 1/4 inch piece of ginger, peeled
- 1 lemon, juiced
- 1/2 cup of water or coconut water

Instructions

1. Wash all the vegetables and the apple thoroughly to remove any pesticides and impurities.
2. Core the apple and chop it into pieces that will easily blend.
3. Peel the ginger and chop it into smaller pieces.
4. Juice the lemon and set the juice aside.
5. In a blender, combine the kale, apple, cucumber, and ginger.
6. Add the lemon juice and water or coconut water to help the ingredients blend smoothly.

7. Blend on high until the mixture becomes a smooth, vibrant green juice.
8. If the juice is too thick, add a bit more water or coconut water to reach your desired consistency.
9. Serve immediately for the best taste and nutrient retention.

Variations

- Add a stalk of celery for extra hydration and a boost in anti-inflammatory properties.

- For a sweeter juice, add another green apple or a small amount of natural sweetener like stevia.

Storage tips

This juice is best enjoyed fresh, but if you need to store it, keep it in an airtight container in the refrigerator for up to 24 hours. It's normal for natural separation to occur, so just give it a good shake before drinking.

Tips for allergens

- For those with allergies to citrus, omit the lemon juice or replace it with a small amount of apple cider vinegar for a similar detoxifying effect.

- Ensure all ingredients are organic to minimize exposure to pesticides, especially important for those undergoing cancer treatment.

Scientific references

- A study published in the *Journal of Nutritional Biochemistry* found that kale contains high levels of antioxidants and phytochemicals that may help prevent certain types of cancer.

- Research in the *International Journal of Preventive Medicine* shows that ginger has anti-inflammatory and antioxidative properties, making it beneficial in the prevention and treatment of cancer.

18. Kale and Sage Stir-Fry

Beneficial effects

This Kale and Sage Stir-Fry is a robust dish designed to bolster the body's natural defenses against cancer. Kale, a leafy green rich in various antioxidants and phytonutrients, supports overall health and can contribute to cancer prevention. Sage is known to contain polyphenols, which have strong antioxidant and anti-inflammatory effects that help combat cancer cells. Together, kale and sage offer a synergistic blend that not only nourishes the body but also aids in the prevention and healing processes of cancer.

Portions	Preparation time	Cooking time
4 servings	10 minutes	15 minutes

Ingredients

- 1 tablespoon olive oil
- 4 cups of chopped kale
- 1 teaspoon ground sage
- 1/4 teaspoon salt
- 1/2 cup Brazil nuts, chopped (optional, for added crunch)
- 1 tablespoon soy sauce
- 1 teaspoon pure agave syrup
- 1/2 cup water
- 1 tablespoon sesame seeds (for garnish)

Instructions

1. Heat the olive oil in a large skillet over medium heat.
2. Add the chopped kale to the skillet and stir-fry for about 5 minutes, until it starts to wilt and become tender.
3. Sprinkle the ground sage and salt over the kale. Stir well to ensure the kale is evenly coated with the spices.
4. Continue to stir-fry the kale for another 2 minutes.
5. Mix the soy sauce, agave syrup, and water in a small bowl, then pour over the kale.
6. Cover the skillet and let the kale simmer for about 5 minutes, or until it is fully tender and the sauce has slightly thickened.

7. Remove from heat and sprinkle with sesame seeds and chopped Brazil nuts over the top before serving.

Variations

- Include other Dr. Sebi-approved vegetables like bell peppers or zucchini for additional nutrients and flavors.

- Replace soy sauce with coconut aminos for those with soy allergies.

Storage tips

Store any leftovers in an airtight container in the refrigerator for up to 3 days. Reheat gently in a skillet or microwave, adding a little water if necessary to prevent drying out.

Tips for allergens

- For those with nut allergies, omit the Brazil nuts or substitute them with suitable seeds such as hemp seeds.

- Ensure that all ingredients used are free from additives that might trigger allergies.

Scientific references

- Research in the *Journal of Medicinal Chemistry* discusses the benefits of phytonutrients found in kale.

19. Mushroom and Nopales Soup

Beneficial effects

This mushroom and nopales Soup utilizes the nutrient density of mushrooms and the unique benefits of nopales to create a comforting dish that may help in the fight against cancer. Nopales are rich in fiber and antioxidants, supporting the immune system, while mushrooms continue to offer antioxidants and beta-glucans. This combination makes the soup not only a delicious meal but also a potential ally in maintaining overall health and well-being.

Portions	Preparation time	Cooking time
4 servings	15 minutes	30 minutes

Ingredients

- 1 tablespoon olive oil
- 1 onion, diced
- 1 pound mixed mushrooms (but not shitake), sliced
- 1 cup nopales, cleaned and diced
- 1 cup turnip greens, roughly chopped
- 4 cups vegetable broth
- 1 teaspoon dried thyme
- Salt to taste
- 1 tablespoon lemon juice

Instructions

1. Heat the olive oil in a large pot over medium heat. Add the diced onion, sautéing until translucent and fragrant, about 5 minutes.
2. Add the sliced mushrooms and nopales to the pot, cooking until the mushrooms are soft and have released their moisture, about 10 minutes.
3. Stir in the turnip greens and pour in the vegetable broth, bringing the mixture to a simmer.
4. Add dried thyme, and season with salt and pepper to taste.
5. Allow the soup to simmer for about 15 minutes, letting the flavors meld together.
6. Just before serving, stir in the lemon juice for a bright burst of flavor.

7. Ladle the soup into bowls and serve hot.

Variations

- For a creamier texture, blend half of the soup until smooth, then mix it back into the pot.

- Add a splash of coconut milk for a richer texture.

- Include additional herbs like oregano or basil for enhanced flavor.

Storage tips

Store any leftover soup in an airtight container in the refrigerator for up to 3 days. Reheat on the stove over medium heat until warmed through.

Tips for allergens

- For those with allergies to certain types of mushrooms, feel free to use only those varieties that are safe for you.

- Ensure the vegetable broth is gluten-free if necessary.

Scientific references

- Research highlighted by *Cancer Research UK* discusses the role of mushrooms in supporting the immune system and their potential use in cancer treatment protocols.

20. Carrot and Ginger Smoothie

Beneficial effects

The carrot and ginger smoothie is a vibrant, nutrient-packed drink that supports overall health, with a particular focus on cancer prevention. Carrots are rich in beta-carotene, a powerful antioxidant that can help reduce the risk of various types of cancer, including lung, breast, and colon cancers. Ginger, known for its anti-inflammatory and antioxidant properties, can help in reducing inflammation and the side effects of cancer treatments. Together, these ingredients create a smoothie that not only boosts your immune system but also aids in detoxifying the body and promoting cellular health.

Portions	Preparation time
2 servings	10 minutes

Ingredients

- 2 large carrots, peeled and chopped
- 1 inch piece of ginger, peeled
- 1 apple (preferably not Granny Smith or Red Delicious), cored and sliced
- 1/2 banana, for sweetness
- 1 cup of water
- Ice cubes (optional)

Instructions

1. Place the chopped carrots, peeled ginger, sliced apple, and banana into a blender.
2. Add water to the blender to help the ingredients blend smoothly.
3. Blend on high speed until the mixture becomes smooth. If the smoothie is too thick, add more water until you reach your desired consistency.
4. Add ice cubes to the blender and pulse a few more times if you prefer a colder smoothie.
5. Pour the smoothie into glasses and serve immediately.

Variations

- To enhance the smoothie's nutritional profile, include a handful of kale; it won't significantly alter the taste but will increase the vitamin and mineral content.

- If you prefer a sweeter smoothie, add 1/4 teaspoon of date sugar.

Storage tips

This smoothie is best enjoyed fresh to maximize the benefits of its nutrients. However, if you need to store it, keep it in an airtight container in the refrigerator for up to 24 hours. Shake well before drinking, as separation may occur.

Tips for allergens

- If you're sensitive to bananas, you can substitute it with mango or peaches for sweetness without affecting the smoothie's health benefits.

Scientific references

- Research in the *International Journal of Preventive Medicine* highlights ginger's potential in reducing inflammation and oxidative stress, which are linked to various chronic diseases, including cancer.

MANAGING INFLAMMATORY CONDITIONS

Inflammation is the body's natural response to injury or infection, a protective mechanism designed to heal and restore. However, when inflammation becomes chronic, it can lead to a myriad of health issues, ranging from arthritis to heart disease, and even cancer. Understanding the dual nature of inflammation—as both a healing process and a potential threat when it becomes chronic—is crucial in managing and preventing inflammatory conditions. Dr. Sebi's approach to tackling inflammation hinges on the principle that the foods we consume can significantly influence our body's inflammatory response. By adopting an alkaline diet rich in plant-based, nutrient-dense foods, one can effectively reduce inflammation and promote healing.

The cornerstone of managing inflammatory conditions according to Dr. Sebi lies in the consumption of anti-inflammatory foods and herbs. These include leafy greens, nuts, seeds, and fruits that are high in antioxidants and minerals, which help neutralize harmful free radicals in the body, thereby reducing inflammation. Foods such as ginger are renowned for their anti-inflammatory properties and play a pivotal role in Dr. Sebi's dietary recommendations. Incorporating these foods into one's diet not only assists in reducing inflammation but also supports overall health and well-being.

Dr. Sebi's recommendations extend beyond mere dietary adjustments; he emphasizes the importance of detoxification in managing inflammation. Through fasting and the consumption of herbal teas, one can cleanse the body of toxins that contribute to inflammation. This detoxification process is integral to restoring the body's natural alkaline state, which is less conducive to inflammation. Dr. Sebi's herbal compounds, specifically designed to cleanse and nourish the body, are instrumental in this process. These herbal remedies, coupled with a strict adherence to an alkaline diet, form the bedrock of his approach to combating inflammatory conditions.

Moreover, Dr. Sebi advocates for a holistic approach to health, where managing stress and maintaining a balance between physical and mental well-being are seen as essential components in the fight against inflammation. Stress is a known trigger for inflammation, and by adopting practices such as meditation, yoga, and deep breathing exercises, one can mitigate stress and its inflammatory effects on the body. This holistic approach underscores the interconnectedness of mind and body, and the importance of nurturing both to achieve a state of health that is free from inflammation.

In the realm of natural healing, the management of inflammatory conditions is not merely about suppressing symptoms but addressing the root causes of inflammation. Through dietary changes, detoxification, and a holistic approach to wellness, one can effectively manage and prevent inflammatory conditions. Dr. Sebi's teachings provide a blueprint for achieving this, advocating for a return to nature and the adoption of a lifestyle that supports the body's natural healing processes. As we delve deeper into the specifics of anti-inflammatory foods and herbs, and explore the practical applications of Dr. Sebi's recommendations, it becomes evident that the key to managing inflammation lies in embracing a lifestyle that is aligned with the principles of natural healing and wellness.

Embracing a lifestyle that minimizes inflammation involves more than just dietary changes; it's about creating a holistic environment for the body to thrive. Dr. Sebi's guidance on incorporating anti-inflammatory foods and herbs into one's diet is a critical step, but equally important is understanding the role of hydration and physical activity in managing inflammation. Drinking ample amounts of alkaline water, ideally enhanced with lemon or lime to further alkalize the body, helps flush out toxins that can contribute to inflammation. Similarly, engaging in regular, moderate exercise boosts circulation and aids in detoxification, both of which are essential in reducing inflammatory responses.

The significance of a clean living environment cannot be overstated when it comes to managing inflammatory conditions. Exposure to pollutants, whether chemical, in the air, or in personal care products, can trigger inflammatory responses. Adopting natural, non-toxic household and personal care products aligns with Dr. Sebi's philosophy of reducing the body's toxic burden. This shift not only helps in managing inflammation, but also supports overall health and aligns with a more sustainable, earth-friendly way of living.

Sleep plays a pivotal role in managing inflammation. Quality sleep allows the body to repair and regenerate, reducing the risk of inflammation-driven diseases. Dr. Sebi recognized the importance of rest and recommended practices that support a good night's sleep, such as establishing a regular sleep schedule, creating a restful environment, and avoiding stimulants before bedtime.

The power of community and positive relationships in healing cannot be underestimated. Social support and engaging in meaningful relationships contribute to emotional well-being, which in turn can reduce stress levels and the inflammatory response associated with chronic stress. Dr. Sebi's holistic approach to health emphasizes the importance of nurturing not just the physical body, but also the mind and spirit through connections with others.

Finally, embracing a mindset of mindfulness and gratitude has profound effects on managing inflammation. Practices such as meditation, journaling, and spending time in nature can help cultivate a state of mental and emotional well-being that supports the body's healing processes. Dr. Sebi encouraged a deep connection with nature as a source of healing energy and a way to ground oneself, reducing the impact of stress and inflammation.

Incorporating these practices into daily life, along with a diet rich in anti-inflammatory foods and herbs, offers a comprehensive approach to managing inflammatory conditions. Dr. Sebi's teachings provide a foundation for a lifestyle that not only addresses the symptoms of inflammation but also targets its root causes, promoting a state of health that is in harmony with the natural world. Through this holistic approach, individuals can empower themselves to take control of their health, reducing their reliance on conventional medicine and embracing the healing power of nature.

Understanding Inflammation and Its Causes

Inflammation is the body's natural defense mechanism against infections, injuries, and toxins, aiming to eliminate harmful stimuli and initiate the healing process. However, when inflammation persists beyond the necessary period, it transitions from being a protective response to a chronic condition that can underlie numerous health issues. Chronic inflammation is at the heart of many diseases, including arthritis, cardiovascular diseases, diabetes, and certain cancers. It's crucial to distinguish between acute inflammation, a short-term response characterized by redness, warmth, swelling, and pain, and chronic inflammation, which is a long-term physiological response that can silently affect the body without overt symptoms.

The causes of chronic inflammation are multifaceted and can stem from various sources. Unhealthy dietary habits, such as the consumption of excessive sugar, refined carbohydrates, and trans fats, contribute significantly to the development of inflammation. These foods can lead to an imbalance in the body's natural flora, increased gut permeability, and ultimately, an inflammatory response. Additionally, environmental factors like exposure to pollutants, industrial chemicals, and secondhand smoke are known triggers of chronic inflammation. Lifestyle factors, including chronic stress, obesity, and sedentary behavior, further exacerbate the body's inflammatory response, creating a cycle that is hard to break without targeted lifestyle changes.

Another critical aspect of inflammation involves the body's immune response. In some cases, the immune system mistakenly attacks healthy tissues, mistaking them for harmful pathogens, leading to autoimmune diseases characterized by chronic inflammation. Conditions such as rheumatoid arthritis, lupus, and inflammatory bowel disease are examples where the immune system's inappropriate response results in persistent inflammation.

Genetic factors also play a role in determining an individual's susceptibility to chronic inflammation. Certain genes can make individuals more prone to inflammatory responses, affecting how their bodies react to external and internal triggers. Understanding these genetic predispositions can be key in developing personalized approaches to managing inflammation.

The gut microbiome, the complex community of microorganisms living in the digestive tract, has emerged as a significant player in the regulation of inflammation. An imbalance in the gut microbiota, known as dysbiosis, can lead to increased permeability of the intestinal lining, often referred to as "leaky gut." This condition allows bacterial endotoxins to enter the bloodstream, triggering systemic inflammation. A diet rich in fiber, fermented foods, and diverse plant-based foods can support a healthy gut microbiome, thereby reducing inflammation.

Addressing chronic inflammation requires a holistic approach that encompasses dietary changes, lifestyle modifications, and, in some cases, medical intervention. Reducing the intake of inflammatory foods and increasing the consumption of anti-inflammatory foods, such as those rich in omega-3 fatty acids, antioxidants, and phytonutrients, is foundational. Regular physical activity, stress management techniques, and ensuring adequate sleep are equally important in mitigating the inflammatory response. In some instances, healthcare professionals may recommend medications or supplements to help manage inflammation, always considering the individual's overall health and specific needs.

In conclusion, understanding the causes and mechanisms of inflammation is crucial in developing effective strategies for prevention and management. By recognizing the factors that contribute to chronic inflammation, individuals can take proactive steps towards improving their health and reducing the risk of inflammation-related diseases. Adopting a lifestyle that supports the body's natural healing processes, prioritizing a balanced diet, regular exercise, stress reduction, and adequate sleep, forms the cornerstone of managing inflammation and enhancing overall well-being.

Anti-Inflammatory Foods and Herbs

Incorporating anti-inflammatory foods and herbs into your diet is a powerful way to combat inflammation and promote overall health. Foods rich in antioxidants, omega-3 fatty acids, and phytonutrients can significantly reduce the body's inflammatory response, offering protection against a range of chronic diseases. Among the most potent anti-inflammatory foods are berries like blueberries and strawberries, which are high in antioxidants and flavonoids. These compounds help reduce inflammation and lower the risk of disease.

Leafy green vegetables, including kale and collards, are packed with vitamins, minerals, and antioxidants. These nutrients work together to combat inflammation and protect the body from the harmful effects of oxidative stress. Nuts, especially walnuts, are another great addition to an anti-inflammatory diet. They are high in vitamin E, magnesium, and healthy fats, all of which have anti-inflammatory properties.

In addition to these foods, certain herbs and spices are renowned for their anti-inflammatory benefits. Ginger is another spice with strong anti-inflammatory and antioxidant properties. It can be consumed fresh, powdered, or as a tea to help reduce inflammation and soothe digestive issues.

Similarly, green tea is packed with antioxidants, including epigallocatechin gallate (EGCG), which has been shown to reduce inflammation and prevent cell damage.

Adopting a diet that emphasizes these anti-inflammatory foods and herbs can lead to noticeable improvements in health. It's not just about adding a few key ingredients to your meals; it's about making a comprehensive shift towards a diet that supports your body's natural ability to fight inflammation. This means reducing the intake of processed foods, sugars, and trans fats, which can trigger inflammatory responses in the body. Instead, focus on whole, nutrient-dense foods that provide a variety of vitamins, minerals, and antioxidants.

For those looking to further embrace the healing power of nature, incorporating herbal teas and supplements can complement an anti-inflammatory diet. However, it's important to consult with a healthcare provider before starting any new supplement, especially for individuals with existing health conditions or those taking medication.

Embracing an anti-inflammatory lifestyle goes beyond diet alone. Regular physical activity, adequate hydration, stress management, and quality sleep are all crucial components of reducing inflammation and promoting overall well-being. By making these holistic changes, individuals can harness the power of natural foods and herbs to support their health and combat inflammation, aligning with Dr. Sebi's teachings on the healing power of nature and the importance of a holistic approach to wellness.

Dr. Sebi's Recommendations for Inflammation

Dr. Sebi's holistic approach to combating inflammation emphasizes the significance of a plant-based, alkaline diet, rich in nutrients and minerals that support the body's natural healing processes. Central to his recommendations is the understanding that inflammation, while a natural response to injury or infection, can become detrimental when it turns chronic, leading to a host of diseases. To counteract this, Dr. Sebi proposed a dietary regimen that not only reduces inflammation but also addresses its underlying causes, promoting overall health and well-being.

At the heart of Dr. Sebi's dietary recommendations for managing inflammation is the consumption of alkaline foods. These include a variety of leafy greens, fruits, nuts, and seeds, all of which contribute to reducing the body's acidic load and fostering an alkaline environment conducive to healing. Specifically, vegetables such as kale, cucumbers, and avocados, and fruits like apples, berries, and melons are encouraged for their high mineral content and alkalizing effects. These foods are not only nutrient-dense but also rich in antioxidants, which play a crucial role in neutralizing free radicals and reducing oxidative stress, a key factor in the inflammatory process.

In addition to emphasizing alkaline foods, Dr. Sebi recommended the inclusion of powerful anti-inflammatory herbs in one's diet. Herbs such as burdock root, dandelion, and elderberry are celebrated for their detoxifying properties and their ability to support liver function, a critical aspect of reducing inflammation. These herbs can be consumed in various forms, including teas and supplements, providing a natural means of cleansing the body and enhancing its healing capabilities.

Another cornerstone of Dr. Sebi's approach to inflammation involves the elimination of mucus-forming foods from the diet. According to Dr. Sebi, foods such as dairy, meat, and processed grains contribute to the accumulation of mucus in the body, exacerbating inflammatory conditions. By removing these foods and replacing them with whole, plant-based alternatives, individuals can significantly reduce inflammation and improve their overall health.

Dr. Sebi also recognized the importance of hydration in managing inflammation. He advocated for the consumption of alkaline water, which helps to flush toxins from the body and maintain a balanced pH level. This, combined with a diet rich in water-dense fruits and vegetables, ensures adequate hydration and supports the body's natural detoxification processes.

Physical activity and stress management are also integral components of Dr. Sebi's recommendations for reducing inflammation. Regular, gentle exercise such as walking, yoga, or swimming helps to improve circulation and facilitate the removal of toxins, while practices such as meditation and deep breathing exercises can significantly reduce stress levels, further mitigating the inflammatory response.

By adopting these dietary and lifestyle changes, individuals can effectively manage inflammation and foster a state of health that aligns with the body's natural rhythms and healing capabilities. Dr. Sebi's teachings offer a path to wellness that is rooted in the wisdom of nature, advocating for a life that is in harmony with the earth and its abundant healing resources. Through a commitment to this holistic approach, it is possible to not only reduce inflammation but also enhance vitality and well-being, embodying the principles of natural healing and the power of an alkaline, plant-based diet.

ADDRESSING KIDNEY DISEASES

Kidney diseases often go unnoticed until they have progressed significantly because the kidneys can perform their job with as little as 20% of their capacity. This silent progression underscores the importance of adopting a lifestyle that supports kidney health, especially in a world where diet and lifestyle choices can put these vital organs under strain. Dr. Sebi's approach to healing kidney diseases focuses on natural, plant-based remedies and an alkaline diet to cleanse and rejuvenate the kidneys, restoring their function and preventing further damage.

The kidneys are responsible for filtering waste products from the blood and excreting them through urine. They also play a crucial role in regulating blood pressure, electrolyte balance, and red blood cell production. When the kidneys are compromised, toxins and excess fluids can build up in the body, leading to swelling, hypertension, and a decline in overall health. Dr. Sebi believed that a diet high in acidic foods and low in minerals stresses the kidneys, leading to inflammation and disease. Conversely, an alkaline diet rich in minerals and antioxidants can help to heal and protect the kidneys.

To support kidney health, Dr. Sebi recommended eliminating acidic, processed foods from the diet and focusing on whole, natural foods that promote an alkaline environment within the body. Essential alkaline foods include leafy green vegetables, cucumbers, avocados, bell peppers, and fruits like apples, berries, and melons. These foods not only support kidney function, but also provide the body with vital nutrients and antioxidants that combat inflammation and disease.

Hydration is another key component of kidney health. Drinking plenty of spring water helps to flush toxins from the kidneys and maintain optimal function. Dr. Sebi advised against consuming tap water due to potential contaminants and instead recommended natural spring water, which is rich in minerals and supports the body's alkaline state.

Herbs play a significant role in Dr. Sebi's approach to treating kidney diseases. Herbs such as dandelion, burdock root, and nettle are known for their diuretic properties, which promote urine production and help to flush out waste products from the kidneys. These herbs also contain antioxidants and compounds that reduce inflammation and support the healing of kidney tissues. Consuming these herbs in the form of teas or supplements can provide a powerful boost to kidney health.

In addition to dietary changes, Dr. Sebi emphasized the importance of lifestyle adjustments in supporting kidney health. Regular exercise helps to lower blood pressure and maintain a healthy weight, both of which are crucial for preventing strain on the kidneys. Stress management techniques such as meditation, deep breathing exercises, and spending time in nature can also help to reduce the risk of kidney disease by lowering stress levels and promoting overall well-being.

For those already suffering from kidney diseases, Dr. Sebi's approach offers a holistic pathway to healing. By adopting an alkaline diet, staying hydrated, using medicinal herbs, and making positive lifestyle changes, individuals can support their kidney health and improve their quality of life. It's important to remember that these natural remedies should complement, not replace, the treatment and advice of healthcare professionals. Working closely with a healthcare provider ensures that any underlying conditions are properly managed and that the natural approach to kidney health is safe and effective.

By embracing Dr. Sebi's principles, individuals can take proactive steps toward preventing and healing kidney diseases naturally. This approach not only supports kidney function but also promotes a healthier, more balanced lifestyle that benefits the entire body.

Overview of Kidney Function and Diseases

Kidneys, two bean-shaped organs located just below the rib cage on either side of the spine, play a pivotal role in maintaining overall health. Their primary function is to filter and remove waste products and excess fluids from the blood through the urine. Beyond waste elimination, kidneys are instrumental in regulating blood pressure, ensuring electrolyte balance, and stimulating the production of red blood cells.

Kidney diseases, often silent in their initial stages, can significantly impair these vital functions. The progression of kidney disease can lead to the accumulation of toxins and fluids in the body, resulting in swelling, high blood pressure, and a decline in health. Chronic kidney disease (CKD), a condition characterized by the gradual loss of kidney function over time, and acute kidney injury (AKI), a sudden loss of kidney function, are among the most prevalent kidney-related health issues.

Factors contributing to kidney disease include diabetes, high blood pressure, recurrent kidney infections, and prolonged obstruction of the urinary tract. Lifestyle choices such as a diet high in processed foods and low in nutrients can also stress the kidneys, leading to inflammation and increased risk of disease.

Preventing kidney disease involves adopting a healthy lifestyle that supports kidney function. This includes maintaining a diet rich in fruits, vegetables, and whole grains to help keep the body's pH levels balanced and reduce the workload on the kidneys. Staying well-hydrated by drinking plenty of water is crucial for helping the kidneys flush out toxins. Regular exercise, managing blood pressure and sugar levels, and avoiding substances that can harm the kidneys, such as NSAIDs and certain antibiotics, are also key preventive measures.

For those already experiencing kidney issues, early detection through regular screening can be lifesaving, especially for individuals with risk factors like diabetes or high blood pressure. Treatment for kidney disease typically focuses on managing the underlying conditions that are contributing to kidney damage. In more advanced cases, dialysis or kidney transplantation may become necessary to perform the functions of the kidneys.

The importance of kidney health cannot be overstated, as these organs are central to the body's ability to detoxify and purify the blood, regulate vital functions, and support overall well-being. By understanding the role of the kidneys and the impact of kidney diseases, individuals can take proactive steps to protect these essential organs and enhance their health naturally, in line with Dr. Sebi's holistic approach to wellness.

Dr. Sebi's Approach to Healing the Kidneys

Dr. Sebi's approach to healing the kidneys revolves around the principle that a natural, plant-based diet rich in alkaline foods, coupled with specific herbs and lifestyle changes, can cleanse, rejuvenate, and restore kidney function. The kidneys, vital organs for filtering waste from the blood and maintaining the body's fluid and electrolyte balance, thrive in an alkaline environment. When the body's pH leans towards acidity due to poor dietary choices and lifestyle habits, it can lead to inflammation and disease in the kidneys. By shifting to an alkaline diet, one can significantly reduce the strain on these organs, promoting healing and better function.

The foundation of Dr. Sebi's kidney health protocol is the elimination of acidic, processed foods and the incorporation of whole, natural foods that foster an alkaline internal environment. Key components of this diet include consuming a variety of leafy green vegetables such as kale and arugula, which are not only alkaline but also rich in essential minerals and antioxidants that support kidney health. Fruits like berries, apples, and melons, despite their natural sugars, contribute to alkalinity and provide hydration, which is crucial for flushing toxins through the kidneys. Avocados, cucumbers, and bell peppers are other staples, offering a wealth of nutrients while helping maintain the body's optimal pH balance.

Hydration plays a critical role in kidney health, with Dr. Sebi emphasizing the importance of drinking ample amounts of spring water throughout the day. This natural water is preferred for its mineral content and purity, aiding in the elimination of waste products and supporting overall kidney function. Additionally, reducing the intake of caffeine and alcohol, which can dehydrate the body and increase the kidneys' workload, is advised to protect these organs.

Herbal remedies are central to Dr. Sebi's approach, with several key herbs identified for their diuretic and healing properties. Dandelion, burdock root, and nettle are particularly beneficial for the kidneys, helping to stimulate urine production, flush out toxins, and reduce inflammation. These herbs can be consumed as teas or supplements, providing a natural means to support kidney cleansing and repair.

Lifestyle adjustments complement the dietary and herbal interventions in Dr. Sebi's kidney healing protocol. Regular, moderate exercise helps to manage blood pressure and body weight, both of which are important for maintaining healthy kidney function. Stress management techniques such as meditation, yoga, and spending time in nature are encouraged to reduce the negative impact of stress on the kidneys. Adequate rest and sleep are also crucial, as they allow the body to heal and regenerate.

By adopting Dr. Sebi's holistic approach to kidney health, individuals can take proactive steps toward preventing and addressing kidney diseases. This natural pathway emphasizes the body's ability to heal itself when supported with the right nutrients, hydration, and lifestyle choices. It's important to note that while these natural remedies can significantly benefit kidney health, they should be used in conjunction with regular medical care, especially for those with existing kidney conditions. Consulting with a healthcare provider before making significant changes to diet or health routines ensures that these natural approaches are safe and effective for each individual's unique health needs.

Herbs and Diet for Kidney Health

Focusing on kidney health through diet and herbs is a transformative approach that aligns with Dr. Sebi's teachings on natural healing. The kidneys, vital organs for filtering waste and balancing fluids in the body, thrive on a diet that minimizes stress and maximizes nutritional support. Embracing an alkaline diet rich in fruits, vegetables, and specific herbs can significantly enhance kidney function and overall well-being.

Leafy green vegetables such as kale and chard are foundational to kidney health. These greens are not only alkaline but also packed with essential minerals like magnesium and potassium, which support the kidneys' natural detoxification processes. Including a variety of these vegetables in your daily meals can help maintain an optimal balance of electrolytes and hydration in the body.

Fruits play a crucial role in a kidney-supportive diet. Berries, cherries, and apples are particularly beneficial due to their high antioxidant content and low potassium levels, making them ideal for those needing to manage their potassium intake. These fruits help combat oxidative stress and inflammation, two factors that can impair kidney function over time.

Whole grains like quinoa, amaranth, and wild rice are excellent sources of B vitamins and fiber, essential for maintaining kidney health. Unlike processed grains, these whole grains do not contribute to acidity or inflammation in the body, supporting the kidneys' ability to filter and eliminate waste efficiently.

Hydration is paramount for kidney health, and spring water is highly recommended for its purity and mineral content. Drinking adequate amounts of water daily helps flush toxins through the kidneys, preventing the buildup of waste and supporting overall kidney function. Herbal teas, particularly those made from kidney-supporting herbs, can also be a beneficial addition to your hydration routine.

Several herbs are known for their diuretic and cleansing properties, making them powerful allies for kidney health. Dandelion root, for example, is a natural diuretic that helps eliminate excess fluid from the body, reducing the strain on the kidneys. Nettle leaf is rich in antioxidants and has been shown to support kidney detoxification and blood purification. Burdock root is another herb celebrated for its blood-cleansing properties and its ability to remove toxins through the urinary tract. Incorporating these herbs into your diet through teas or supplements can provide a significant boost to kidney health.

It's also important to limit the intake of foods that can stress the kidneys. High-sodium foods, processed meats, and foods high in animal protein can increase the burden on the kidneys, leading to potential issues over time. By focusing on plant-based, whole foods and minimizing the consumption of processed and high-sodium foods, you can support your kidneys and promote their health and longevity.

Adopting a lifestyle that includes regular exercise and stress reduction techniques further supports kidney health. Physical activity helps maintain healthy blood pressure and weight, both of which are important for kidney function. Stress management practices like meditation, yoga, and deep breathing exercises can help mitigate the negative effects of stress on the kidneys.

By integrating these dietary and lifestyle changes, individuals can take proactive steps toward maintaining healthy kidneys. Emphasizing alkaline foods, hydrating properly, and incorporating beneficial herbs into your diet are key components of Dr. Sebi's approach to natural healing. This holistic pathway not only supports kidney health but also promotes a balanced and healthy lifestyle that can prevent disease and enhance overall well-being. Remember, while these natural approaches offer numerous benefits, it's important to consult with a healthcare provider before making significant changes, especially for those with existing kidney conditions or other health concerns.

4 Recipes for Healing Kidney Diseases

21. Nettle and Dandelion Tea

Beneficial effects

Nettle and dandelion tea is a natural diuretic that helps cleanse the kidneys, remove toxins, and improve kidney function. Both nettle and dandelion are rich in nutrients and antioxidants, which can reduce inflammation, combat infection, and support overall kidney health. This herbal tea is particularly beneficial for those dealing with kidney diseases, as it aids in flushing out waste materials and excess fluid from the body, reducing the burden on the kidneys.

Portions	Preparation time	Cooking time
2 servings	10 minutes	5-10 minutes

Ingredients

- 1 tablespoon dried nettle leaves
- 1 tablespoon dried dandelion leaves
- 4 cups of water
- Lemon (optional, for taste)

Instructions

1. Bring the water to a boil in a medium-sized pot.
2. Add the dried nettle and dandelion leaves to the boiling water.
3. Reduce the heat and let it simmer for 5 to 10 minutes, allowing the herbs to steep and their beneficial compounds to infuse into the water.
4. Strain the tea into cups or a teapot, discarding the leaves.
5. If desired, add lemon to taste for added flavor.
6. Enjoy the tea warm, ideally drinking one cup in the morning and another in the evening for best results.

Variations

- For an added detox effect, include a slice of fresh ginger in the tea while it simmers.
- Mix in a cinnamon stick during the simmering process for a warming, spicy flavor.
- Combine with peppermint leaves for a refreshing twist.

Storage tips

If you have leftover tea, it can be stored in the refrigerator for up to 2 days. Reheat gently on the stove or enjoy chilled for a refreshing drink.

Tips for allergens

- For those with allergies to plants in the Asteraceae family, such as dandelions, consider substituting with another kidney-supportive herb (but not parsley, which is prohibited in this diet).

22. Raspberry and Lemon Juice

Beneficial effects

Raspberry and Lemon Juice is a refreshing and potent drink aimed at supporting kidney health and preventing urinary tract infections (UTIs). Raspberries are rich in nutrients and antioxidants, known for their anti-inflammatory properties and ability to promote overall urinary tract health. Lemon juice, rich in vitamin C, enhances the body's immune response and aids in detoxification processes. Together, they create a powerful beverage that not only promotes kidney health but also helps maintain a balanced urinary tract environment.

Portions	Preparation time
2 servings	5 minutes

Ingredients

- 1 cup of fresh raspberries
- 2 tablespoons of fresh lemon juice
- 2 cups of water
- Pure agave syrup to taste (optional)

Instructions

1. Rinse the raspberries under cold water and then add them to a blender.
2. Pour in the fresh lemon juice and water.
3. Blend on high until the mixture is smooth.
4. Strain the juice through a fine mesh sieve or cheesecloth into a pitcher or glasses to remove the raspberries pulp.
5. Serve the juice chilled or over ice for a refreshing drink.

Variations

- For an extra detox boost, add a slice of ginger before blending.

Storage tips

This juice is best enjoyed fresh but can be stored in an airtight container in the refrigerator for up to 24 hours. Shake well before serving if separation occurs.

Tips for allergens

- For those with allergies to agave, use date sugar.

- Ensure all ingredients are organic to minimize exposure to pesticides, especially important for those with sensitivities.

Scientific references

- Research highlights the benefits of antioxidants in raspberries, which can support urinary tract health.

- Studies in the *American Journal of Clinical Nutrition* discuss the role of vitamin C, found in lemon juice, in enhancing immune system function and detoxification processes.

23. Basil and Celery Smoothie

Beneficial effects

The Basil and Celery Smoothie is a refreshing and nutritious drink that supports kidney health and detoxification. Basil, known for its anti-inflammatory and antioxidant properties, also acts as a natural detoxifier, aiding in flushing out toxins and reducing the burden on the kidneys. Celery, rich in antioxidants, supports overall kidney function and helps lower blood pressure, a common factor in kidney disease. This smoothie is an excellent way to hydrate and provide your body with essential nutrients for kidney health.

Portions	Preparation time
2 servings	10 minutes

Ingredients

- 1 cup chopped basil
- 2 cups chopped celery
- 1 apple, cored and sliced
- 1/2 cucumber, sliced
- 1 tablespoon lemon juice
- 1 cup water
- Ice cubes (optional)

Instructions

1. Wash the basil and celery thoroughly to remove any dirt or impurities.
2. Place the chopped basil, celery, sliced apple, and cucumber into a blender.
3. Add the lemon juice and water.
4. Blend on high speed until the mixture becomes smooth.
5. If desired, add ice cubes and blend again to chill the smoothie.
6. Serve the smoothie immediately for the freshest taste and best nutrient retention.

Variations

- For a sweeter smoothie, add a teaspoon of pure agave syrup.
- Include a piece of ginger for additional anti-inflammatory benefits.

- Swap out the apple for a pear without significantly altering the taste.

Storage tips

It's best to consume the smoothie immediately after preparation to ensure maximum freshness and effectiveness of the nutrients. If you must store it, keep the smoothie in an airtight container in the refrigerator for up to 24 hours. Shake well before consuming as separation may occur.

Tips for allergens

- For those with allergies to celery, substitute with more cucumber for a green nutrient boost.

- Ensure the water used does not contain added flavors or preservatives that might cause allergic reactions.

24. Burdock Root and Ginger Soup with Basil

Beneficial effects

Burdock root and ginger soup is a warming and detoxifying dish that supports kidney health by promoting the body's natural filtration processes and helping to cleanse the bloodstream. Burdock root is celebrated for its blood-purifying properties and high antioxidant content, which aid in toxin removal. Ginger contributes anti-inflammatory benefits, helping reduce inflammation and supporting overall digestive health. Enhanced with basil, this soup is not only comforting but also a potent tool in maintaining kidney health and function.

Portions	Preparation time	Cooking time
4 servings	15 minutes	1 hour

Ingredients

- 1 tablespoon olive oil
- 1 large onion, chopped
- 2 inches fresh ginger, peeled and grated
- 2 cups burdock root, scrubbed and sliced
- 4 cups vegetable broth
- 2 cups water
- Salt to taste
- Fresh basil, chopped (for garnish)

Instructions

1. Heat the olive oil in a large pot over medium heat. Add the chopped onion and sauté until translucent, about 5 minutes.
2. Add the grated ginger to the pot and cook for another 2 minutes, stirring frequently.
3. Add the sliced burdock root to the pot and sauté for 5 minutes, allowing the burdock root to slightly soften.
4. Pour in the vegetable broth and water, and bring the mixture to a boil.
5. Reduce the heat to low and let the soup simmer, covered, for about 50 minutes or until the burdock root is tender.
6. Season with salt to taste.

7. Serve the soup hot, garnished with fresh chopped basil.

Variations

- Include squash for additional vitamins and a more complex flavor profile.
- For a spicier soup, add a pinch of cayenne pepper.

Storage tips

Store any leftover soup in an airtight container in the refrigerator for up to 3 days. Reheat on the stove over medium heat until warmed through.

Tips for allergens

- Ensure the vegetable broth is free from allergens specific to your dietary needs, such as gluten or soy.

Scientific references

- A study published in the *International Journal of Rheumatic Diseases* found that burdock root has potent antioxidant and anti-inflammatory properties, which can support kidney health and detoxification.

- Research in the *Journal of Ethnopharmacology* highlights ginger's role in reducing inflammation and its therapeutic potential in treating various conditions, including those affecting the kidneys.

TREATING DIGESTIVE ISSUES AND LIVER DETOX

Digestive issues and liver detox are crucial areas when it comes to maintaining optimal health and well-being. A healthy digestive system ensures that your body can absorb all the nutrients it needs while eliminating toxins efficiently. Similarly, a well-functioning liver plays a pivotal role in detoxifying the body, processing nutrients, and supporting overall health. Dr. Sebi's approach to treating digestive issues and liver detox focuses on natural, plant-based diets and herbal remedies that support the body's natural healing processes.

For those struggling with digestive problems, whether it's bloating, irregular bowel movements, or more severe conditions like irritable bowel syndrome (IBS), the key is often to return to a diet that is as close to nature as possible. Dr. Sebi recommended an alkaline diet rich in fruits, vegetables, whole grains, and nuts, all of which support digestive health. Foods like papaya, which contains the enzyme papain, can aid in digestion, while leafy greens help to cleanse the colon. Alkaline water and herbal teas, such as ginger and peppermint, are also beneficial for soothing the digestive system.

When it comes to liver detox, the focus is on foods and herbs that naturally cleanse the liver and enhance its ability to filter toxins from the blood. Dandelion root tea is a powerful herbal remedy that supports liver function by helping to remove toxins and improve bile flow. Burdock root is another herb that not only detoxifies the liver, but also supports kidney health. Incorporating foods high in antioxidants, such as berries, beets, and garlic, can also help protect the liver from damage and support its healing process.

A simple step-by-step guide to starting a liver detox might include:

1. Begin each day with a glass of warm lemon water to stimulate the liver.

2. Incorporate liver-supporting foods into your diet, such as leafy greens, green tea.

3. Drink herbal teas known for their liver-cleansing properties, such as dandelion or milk thistle, twice a day.

4. Avoid processed foods, sugars, and unhealthy fats, which can burden the liver.

5. Stay hydrated with alkaline water throughout the day to help flush toxins from the body.

6. Consider a short juice fast using vegetables like beets and cucumbers to give your liver a break from processing solid foods.

Remember, the objective is not only to cleanse the liver, but to support its health long-term through dietary and lifestyle changes. This might include regular physical activity, reducing stress through practices like meditation or yoga, and ensuring adequate sleep each night.

For those new to these concepts, it's important to start slowly and listen to your body. Sudden, drastic changes to your diet or lifestyle can be overwhelming and counterproductive. Begin by incorporating a few liver-friendly foods and one or two herbal teas into your daily routine, gradually increasing as your body adjusts. Always consult with a healthcare provider before starting any new health regimen, especially if you have existing health conditions or are taking medications.

By adopting Dr. Sebi's principles of natural healing and focusing on an alkaline diet and herbal remedies, you can support your digestive health and liver function. This holistic approach not only addresses specific health issues but also promotes overall well-being, allowing you to lead a healthier, more vibrant life.

Common Digestive Problems and Their Causes

Digestive issues are a widespread concern affecting a significant portion of the population at some point in their lives. These problems can range from mild discomfort to severe conditions that impact daily living and overall health. Understanding the common digestive problems and their causes is the first step towards addressing and managing them effectively.

One of the most prevalent digestive issues is bloating, characterized by a feeling of fullness or swelling in the abdominal area. Bloating can be caused by overeating, eating too quickly, or consuming foods that are hard to digest. Foods high in fat, dairy products, and certain vegetables like cabbage and beans are known to contribute to this condition. Additionally, carbonated drinks can also cause gas to get trapped in the digestive system, leading to bloating.

Constipation is another common digestive problem, defined by infrequent bowel movements or difficulty passing stools. Causes of constipation include a diet low in fiber, insufficient water intake, lack of physical activity, and ignoring the urge to have a bowel movement. Stress and changes in routine can also affect bowel habits, leading to constipation.

On the other end of the spectrum is diarrhea, characterized by loose, watery stools occurring more frequently than usual. Diarrhea can result from infections caused by bacteria, viruses, or parasites, often contracted from contaminated food or water. It can also be a side effect of medications, especially antibiotics, or a symptom of digestive disorders like irritable bowel syndrome (IBS) or inflammatory bowel diseases (IBD) such as Crohn's disease and ulcerative colitis.

Irritable bowel syndrome (IBS) is a chronic condition that affects the large intestine, causing symptoms like cramping, abdominal pain, bloating, gas, and diarrhea or constipation. The exact cause of IBS is unknown, but it's believed to be related to increased sensitivity of the gut, abnormal muscle contractions, and disruptions in the communication between the brain and the digestive system. Stress and certain foods can trigger or worsen IBS symptoms.

Heartburn and acid reflux are conditions that occur when stomach acid flows back into the esophagus, causing irritation and a burning sensation in the chest. These issues are often the result of eating spicy or fatty foods, overeating, or lying down too soon after eating. Obesity, smoking, and certain medications can also increase the risk of developing heartburn and acid reflux.

Gastroesophageal reflux disease (GERD) is a more severe form of acid reflux that can lead to more serious complications if left untreated. GERD occurs when acid reflux happens frequently, leading to inflammation in the esophagus. Factors contributing to GERD include obesity, hiatal hernia, pregnancy, and smoking.

Peptic ulcers are sores that develop on the lining of the stomach, small intestine, or esophagus, caused by the bacteria H. pylori or long-term use of nonsteroidal anti-inflammatory drugs (NSAIDs) like aspirin and ibuprofen. Symptoms include stomach pain, bloating, and indigestion.

Understanding the causes behind these common digestive problems is crucial for identifying the best approaches to treatment and management. Lifestyle changes, such as adjusting diet, increasing physical activity, and managing stress, can significantly improve digestive health. For persistent or severe symptoms, consulting a healthcare provider is essential to rule out more serious conditions and develop an effective treatment plan. Adopting Dr. Sebi's principles of an alkaline diet and natural remedies can also support digestive health by promoting a balanced internal environment conducive to healing and well-being.

Dr. Sebi's Detoxification Methods

Dr. Sebi's detoxification methods are centered around the principle of removing toxins and waste materials from the body to promote healing and restore health. His approach is holistic, focusing on the use of natural, plant-based foods and herbs to cleanse the body's organs and systems. The core of his detoxification process involves an alkaline diet, herbal teas, fasting, and hydration, all aimed at enhancing the body's natural ability to heal itself.

The alkaline diet is fundamental to Dr. Sebi's detoxification method. This diet emphasizes the consumption of electric foods—those that are natural, unprocessed, and rich in minerals to help shift the body's pH towards a more alkaline state. Alkaline foods, such as leafy greens, fruits, nuts, seeds, and alkaline grains, are believed to reduce inflammation, cleanse the body's cells, and support vital organ functions. By eliminating acidic foods, such as processed foods, meats, dairy, and sugar, the body can reduce mucus and inflammation, which are often the root causes of disease.

Herbal teas play a significant role in Dr. Sebi's detoxification process. Herbs like burdock root, dandelion, and sarsaparilla are known for their powerful cleansing properties. These herbs support liver function, aid in the removal of toxins from the blood, and help cleanse the kidneys and lymphatic system. Drinking herbal teas daily, especially those with diuretic properties, can assist in flushing out toxins and promoting hydration.

Fasting is another critical component of Dr. Sebi's detox methods. Periodic fasting allows the body to rest from the constant work of digestion, enabling it to focus on healing and regeneration. During fasting, the consumption of solid foods is minimized or eliminated for a certain period, while hydration is maintained through the intake of alkaline water and herbal teas. This practice can help reset the digestive system, reduce toxin load, and support overall health.

Hydration is essential for effective detoxification. Dr. Sebi emphasized the importance of drinking plenty of alkaline water to help flush toxins from the body. Alkaline water, which has a higher pH level than regular drinking water, is believed to neutralize acid in the bloodstream, leading to improved circulation, detoxification, and nutrient absorption. Staying well-hydrated supports kidney function, aids in digestion, and helps maintain healthy skin.

Implementing Dr. Sebi's detoxification methods into your daily routine can start with simple steps. Begin by gradually incorporating more alkaline foods into your diet and reducing the intake of acidic and processed foods. Start your day with a glass of warm lemon water to stimulate digestion and liver function. Incorporate herbal teas into your daily regimen, focusing on those that support detoxification. Consider practicing short periods of fasting, starting with one day and gradually increasing as your body adjusts. Finally, ensure you are drinking enough alkaline water throughout the day to support the detoxification process.

Remember, the goal of detoxification is not only to remove toxins, but also to nourish the body, support healing, and promote a state of well-being. It's important to listen to your body and make adjustments as needed. Consulting with a healthcare provider before making significant changes to your diet or lifestyle, especially if you have existing health conditions or concerns, is always recommended. By following Dr. Sebi's principles of natural healing and detoxification, you can take meaningful steps toward improving your health and vitality.

Alkaline Foods for Digestive Health

Alkaline foods play a pivotal role in promoting digestive health by creating an environment that nurtures beneficial gut bacteria and ensures efficient digestion and nutrient absorption. The foundation of an alkaline diet for digestive wellness hinges on consuming a variety of fruits, vegetables, nuts, seeds, and whole grains that not only support the body's pH balance, but also provide essential fiber, vitamins, and minerals.

Fruits such as bananas, melons, and avocados are excellent alkaline options that offer a rich source of potassium, a key mineral in maintaining a healthy pH level in the body. These fruits, along with papayas, contain enzymes that aid in breaking down food, making the digestive process smoother and more efficient. Vegetables, especially leafy greens like kale and Swiss chard, are high in magnesium, another crucial component for digestive health, as they help to relax the muscles in the digestive tract, reducing cramping and discomfort.

Quinoa and millet are examples of alkaline grains that provide a hearty source of fiber and nutrients without causing acidity or bloating, common issues associated with more refined grains.

Hydration is another key aspect of supporting digestive health with an alkaline diet. Alkaline water, which has a higher pH level than regular tap water, can help neutralize stomach acidity, reducing symptoms of acid reflux and improving overall digestion. Herbal teas, such as peppermint and chamomile, are not only soothing but also possess properties that can alleviate digestive discomfort and promote a healthy gut.

To integrate these alkaline foods into your diet for optimal digestive health, start by incorporating a variety of fruits and vegetables into each meal, aiming for a colorful plate that ensures a wide range of nutrients. Snack on nuts and seeds, or add them to salads and smoothies for an extra fiber boost. Choose whole grains over refined ones to avoid spikes in blood sugar and potential digestive issues. Finally, ensure you're drinking plenty of alkaline water and herbal teas throughout the day to stay hydrated and support your digestive system.

Remember, transitioning to an alkaline diet for digestive health is a process that should be approached gradually, allowing your body to adjust to the changes. It's also important to listen to your body and observe how different foods affect your digestion, making adjustments as needed to find what works best for you. By focusing on alkaline foods that promote digestive health, you can improve your overall well-being, experiencing fewer digestive issues and enjoying a more vibrant life.

Liver Cleansing Protocols

Liver cleansing protocols are essential in promoting a healthy detoxification process, supporting the liver's ability to filter toxins, and maintaining overall vitality. The liver, a key player in the body's natural detoxification system, processes nutrients from the food we eat, helps to detoxify harmful substances, and plays a critical role in managing the body's metabolism. A healthy liver contributes to better energy levels, improved digestion, and a stronger immune system. To support liver health, incorporating specific foods, herbs, and lifestyle practices into your daily routine can be incredibly beneficial.

Firstly, focusing on a diet rich in whole, plant-based foods is crucial. Foods that are particularly supportive of liver health include leafy greens like kale, which is high in chlorophyll and help to purify the blood, thus aiding the liver in its detoxification efforts.

Herbs play a significant role in liver cleansing protocols. Milk thistle, for example, is widely recognized for its liver-protective qualities. It contains silymarin, a compound that supports liver health by promoting the regeneration of liver cells and protecting against damage from toxins. Dandelion root is another herb that benefits the liver by stimulating bile production, which helps to break down fats and support the detoxification process. Incorporating these herbs into your diet through teas or supplements can provide a significant boost to your liver's health.

Hydration is another key element in supporting liver function. Drinking adequate amounts of water each day helps to flush toxins out of the body, aiding the liver in its vital detoxification role. Adding a slice of lemon to your water can further support liver health, as lemon juice stimulates the liver and aids in the digestion and detoxification process.

Regular physical activity is also beneficial for liver health. Exercise helps to reduce liver fat, decrease inflammation, and increase energy levels. Engaging in activities such as walking, yoga, or cycling can help to maintain a healthy weight and support overall liver function.

To implement a liver cleansing protocol, consider the following steps:

1. Begin your day with a glass of warm lemon water to stimulate the liver and aid digestion.
2. Incorporate liver-supporting foods into your meals, focusing on leafy greens, cruciferous vegetables, and beets.
3. Drink herbal teas such as milk thistle or dandelion root twice daily to support liver health.
4. Ensure you are staying hydrated by drinking at least 8 glasses of water throughout the day.
5. Engage in regular physical activity to support liver function and overall health.

By adopting these practices, you can support your liver's health and enhance its detoxification capabilities. Remember, the liver is a vital organ that plays a crucial role in maintaining the body's overall well-being, and taking steps to support its function can lead to improved health and vitality. Always consult with a healthcare provider before starting any new health regimen, especially if you have existing health conditions or are taking medications.

4 Recipes for Healing Digestive Issues

25. Ginger and Fennel Tea

Beneficial effects
Ginger and fennel tea combines the digestive benefits of ginger, known for its ability to alleviate nausea, bloating, and indigestion, with the soothing properties of fennel, which can help reduce gas and cramping. This tea is an excellent natural remedy for supporting digestive health and providing relief from discomfort associated with digestive issues.

Portions	Preparation time	Cooking time
2 servings	5 minutes	10 minutes

Ingredients
- 1 tablespoon of fresh ginger, grated
- 1 tablespoon of fennel seeds
- 4 cups of water
- Lemon to taste (optional)

Instructions
1. Bring the water to a boil in a medium-sized pot.
2. Add the grated ginger and fennel seeds to the boiling water.
3. Reduce the heat and allow the mixture to simmer for about 10 minutes, letting the flavors infuse.
4. Strain the tea into cups, removing the ginger and fennel seeds.
5. If desired, add lemon to taste for additional flavor.
6. Serve the tea warm, enjoying the soothing and digestive benefits.

Variations
- For a stronger tea, allow the ginger and fennel seeds to simmer for an additional 5 minutes before straining.
- Add a cinnamon stick during simmering for a warming spice flavor.

- Incorporate a peppermint tea bag for a refreshing twist and added digestive benefits.

Storage tips

This tea is best enjoyed fresh, but you can store any leftovers in the refrigerator for up to 2 days. Reheat gently on the stove or enjoy chilled.

Tips for allergens

- Ensure that the fennel seeds are sourced from a supplier that does not process other allergenic foods in the same facility to avoid cross-contamination.

Scientific references

- A study published in the *Journal of Ethnopharmacology* highlights ginger's effectiveness in alleviating symptoms of nausea and indigestion.

- Research in the *Journal of Food Science* discusses the carminative properties of fennel seeds, supporting their use in reducing gas and bloating.

26. Papaya and Mango Smoothie

Beneficial effects

The papaya and mango smoothie is a delightful blend that aids in digestion and supports gastrointestinal health. Papaya contains an enzyme called papain, which helps break down proteins and facilitates natural digestion processes. Mango, though not as rich in digestive enzymes as pineapple, still contributes beneficial nutrients and fiber that aid digestion. Together, these tropical fruits offer a powerful duo to help ease digestive issues, promote nutrient absorption, and soothe the digestive tract.

Portions	Preparation time
2 servings	10 minutes

Ingredients

- 1 cup fresh papaya, cubed
- 1 cup fresh mango, cubed
- 1 banana, sliced
- 1 cup water
- 1/2 teaspoon fresh ginger, grated
- Ice cubes (optional)

Instructions

1. Place the cubed papaya and mango into a blender.
2. Add the sliced banana and grated ginger for an extra digestive boost.
3. Pour in the water to facilitate blending and enhance hydration.
4. Add ice cubes if you prefer a colder smoothie.
5. Blend on high until the mixture becomes smooth and creamy.
6. Serve immediately to enjoy the fresh flavors and digestive benefits.

Variations

- For added protein, include a scoop of your favorite plant-based protein powder.
- For a sweeter smoothie, drizzle in a bit of pure agave syrup to taste.

Storage tips

This smoothie is best enjoyed fresh to maximize the benefits of its active enzymes. However, if you need to store it, keep it in an airtight container in the refrigerator for up to 24 hours. Shake well before consuming as separation may occur.

Tips for allergens

- Ensure the banana and other ingredients are suitable for those with specific food sensitivities or allergies.

Scientific references

- "Papain, a plant enzyme of biological importance: A review," published in the *American Journal of Biochemistry and Biotechnology*, discusses the digestive benefits of papain found in papaya.

- While mango doesn't contain bromelain, it is still valued for its nutritional content and fiber, which support overall digestive health.

27. Chamomile and Peppermint Infusion

Beneficial effects

Chamomile and peppermint infusion is a soothing and calming beverage, perfect for aiding with digestive issues. Chamomile is known for its ability to relax the muscles of the digestive tract, easing cramps and reducing inflammation, which can help alleviate symptoms of indigestion, gas, and bloating. Peppermint, on the other hand, has been shown to relieve symptoms of irritable bowel syndrome (IBS), including discomfort, bloating, and bowel movement irregularities. Together, they create a powerful herbal remedy that not only soothes the stomach, but also promotes overall digestive health.

Portions	Preparation time	Cooking time
2 servings	5 minutes	10 minutes

Ingredients

- 2 tablespoons dried chamomile flowers
- 2 tablespoons dried peppermint leaves
- 4 cups boiling water
- Lemon (optional, for taste)

Instructions

1. Boil 4 cups of water in a kettle or pot.
2. Place the dried chamomile flowers and dried peppermint leaves in a teapot or large heatproof pitcher.
3. Pour the boiling water over the chamomile and peppermint, ensuring all the leaves are submerged.
4. Cover and steep for 10 minutes to allow the herbs to fully infuse their flavors and beneficial properties into the water.
5. Strain the infusion into cups, discarding the used herbs.
6. If desired, add a squeeze of lemon to taste.
7. Enjoy the infusion warm to maximize its soothing effects on the digestive system.

Variations

- For a cooler, refreshing drink, allow the infusion to cool to room temperature, then refrigerate until chilled. Serve over ice.

- Add a slice of ginger during the steeping process for an extra digestive boost and a hint of spice.

- Combine with a cinnamon stick, while steeping for additional warmth and flavor complexity.

Storage tips

If you have leftover infusion, it can be stored in the refrigerator for up to 24 hours. Reheat gently on the stove or enjoy cold for a refreshing herbal drink.

Tips for allergens

- For those with allergies to chamomile or peppermint, consider substituting with ginger tea, which also offers digestive benefits.

Scientific references

- A study published in the *Journal of Clinical Gastroenterology* found that peppermint oil is significantly effective in treating symptoms of irritable bowel syndrome (IBS).

- Research in the *Molecular Medicine Reports* highlights the anti-inflammatory and antispasmodic effects of chamomile, supporting its use in treating digestive discomfort.

28. Aloe Vera and Cucumber Juice

Beneficial effects

Aloe vera and cucumber juice is a refreshing and hydrating drink that supports digestive health and aids in liver detoxification. Aloe vera is known for its natural laxative properties and ability to soothe and protect the gastrointestinal tract, promoting healthy digestion. Cucumber, being high in water content and rich in antioxidants, helps in flushing out toxins from the body and maintaining hydration. Together, they create a powerful detoxifying drink that can help alleviate digestive issues and support overall liver function.

Portions	Preparation time
2 servings	10 minutes

Ingredients

- 1/2 cup of pure aloe vera gel
- 1 large cucumber, peeled and chopped
- 1/2 cup of water or coconut water
- 1 tablespoon of lemon juice
- Pure agave syrup to taste (optional)

Instructions

1. Extract the aloe vera gel from the leaf, if using fresh aloe. Ensure to rinse the gel thoroughly to remove any latex residue.
2. Place the chopped cucumber in a blender.
3. Add the aloe vera gel, water or coconut water, and lemon juice to the blender.
4. Blend on high until the mixture becomes smooth.
5. Taste the juice and, if desired, add pure agave syrup to sweeten.
6. Strain the juice through a fine mesh sieve or cheesecloth into glasses to remove any pulp.
7. Serve the juice immediately, or chill in the refrigerator for a refreshing cold drink.

Variations

- Add a piece of ginger before blending for an extra refreshing taste and additional digestive benefits.

- For a more filling drink, include a green apple or pear in the blend.

- Substitute lemon juice with lime juice for a different citrusy flavor.

Storage tips

This juice is best enjoyed fresh to maximize the benefits of its nutrients. However, if you need to store it, keep it in an airtight container in the refrigerator for up to 24 hours. Shake well before serving as separation may occur.

Tips for allergens

- For those with sensitivities to aloe vera, start with a small amount to ensure it agrees with your digestive system.

- If using store-bought aloe vera gel, ensure it's food-grade and free from additives or aloin.

Scientific references

- "Aloe vera in treatment of refractory irritable bowel syndrome: Trial on Iranian patients" published in the *Journal of Research in Medical Sciences*, highlights the benefits of aloe vera in treating IBS symptoms.

- "Hydration and health: a review" in the *Nutrition Reviews* discusses the importance of hydration for overall health, supporting the inclusion of high-water-content foods like cucumber in the diet.

4 Recipes for Liver Problems

29. Dandelion Root Tea

Beneficial effects

Dandelion root tea is a traditional herbal remedy known for its powerful detoxifying properties. It supports liver function by helping to filter toxins more efficiently, promoting the elimination of waste through increased urine production. Rich in antioxidants, dandelion root tea can also help combat inflammation and protect liver cells from damage. Its mild diuretic effect aids in reducing water retention, making it a beneficial drink for overall liver health.

Portions	Preparation time	Cooking time
2 servings	5 minutes	10 minutes

Ingredients

- 2 tablespoons of dried dandelion root
- 4 cups of water
- Lemon to taste (optional)

Instructions

1. Bring the water to a boil in a medium-sized pot.
2. Add the dried dandelion root to the boiling water.
3. Reduce the heat and simmer for about 10 minutes, allowing the dandelion root to steep and its beneficial compounds to infuse into the water.
4. Strain the tea into cups, discarding the dandelion root.
5. If desired, add lemon to taste for additional flavor.
6. Enjoy the tea warm, ideally in the morning or before meals to maximize its liver-supporting benefits.

Variations

- For a more complex flavor, add a cinnamon stick or a few slices of fresh ginger to the pot while simmering.

- Combine with milk thistle tea for an enhanced liver detox effect.

Storage tips

This tea is best enjoyed fresh, but you can store any leftovers in the refrigerator for up to 2 days. Reheat gently on the stove or enjoy chilled as a refreshing herbal iced tea.

Tips for allergens

- For those with allergies to plants in the Asteraceae family, such as dandelions, start with a small amount to ensure it agrees with your system.

Scientific references

- A study published in the *Journal of Alternative and Complementary Medicine* found that dandelion root extract had a protective effect on liver tissue in the presence of toxic substances.

- Research in the International *Journal of Molecular Sciences* highlights the antioxidant properties of dandelion root and its potential benefits in preventing and treating liver diseases.

30. Liver-Supporting Kale and Walnut Smoothie

Beneficial effects

This potent liver-supporting smoothie leverages the detoxifying properties of kale to help cleanse and rejuvenate the liver. Kale is renowned for its high antioxidant content, including vitamins A, C, and K, which support liver health by protecting liver cells from toxins and promoting their regeneration. Combined with other liver-friendly ingredients, this smoothie is an excellent choice for those looking to support their liver function naturally.

Portions
2 servings

Preparation time
10 minutes

Ingredients

- 2 cups kale leaves, roughly chopped
- 1/2 avocado
- 1/2 banana
- 1 cup water
- 1 tablespoon walnuts
- Ice cubes (optional)

Instructions

1. Place the chopped kale, avocado, and banana into a blender.
2. Add the walnuts and pour in water to facilitate blending.
3. Blend on high speed until the mixture becomes smooth and creamy.
4. For a chilled smoothie, add ice cubes and blend until smooth.
5. Serve immediately for the best taste and nutrient retention.

Variations

- For an extra protein boost, add a scoop of your favorite plant-based protein powder.
- Add a squeeze of lemon or lime juice for a refreshing citrus twist and vitamin C boost.

Storage tips

This smoothie is best enjoyed fresh to ensure the maximum potency of the nutrients' beneficial properties. However, if you need to store it, keep it in an airtight container in the refrigerator for up to 24 hours. Stir well before consuming as separation may occur.

Tips for allergens

- For those with nut allergies, ensure the walnuts used are suitable or omit them entirely if necessary.

- Ensure all ingredients are organic and free from additives or fillers that might cause allergies.

31. Zucchini and Lemon Salad

Beneficial effects

This Zucchini and Lemon Salad is a nutritious dish that supports liver health and detoxification. Zucchini is high in water content and dietary fiber, which aid in digestion and liver function. Avocado adds healthy fats and further supports liver health with its nutrient-rich profile. Lemon, high in vitamin C, enhances detoxification processes and the absorption of antioxidants. Tarragon adds a unique flavor and has properties that may aid digestion and liver health. This salad is not only delicious but also helps in lowering cholesterol levels and improving digestive health.

Portions	Preparation time
4 servings	20 minutes

Ingredients

- 4 large zucchinis, thinly sliced
- 2 lemons, one juiced and one sliced for garnish
- 2 tablespoons extra virgin olive oil
- 1 avocado, diced
- Salt to taste
- A handful of fresh tarragon, chopped

Instructions

1. Fill a large bowl with cold water and add the juice of one lemon.
2. As you slice the zucchini, place them in the lemon water to prevent browning.
3. Drain the zucchinis and pat dry with paper towels.
4. In a large salad bowl, combine the sliced zucchinis, diced avocado, and chopped tarragon.
5. Drizzle with extra virgin olive oil and the remaining lemon juice. Toss to coat evenly.
6. Season with salt to taste.
7. Garnish with lemon slices.
8. Serve immediately or chill in the refrigerator for 30 minutes before serving to enhance the flavors.

Variations

- Include cherry tomatoes or olives for additional color and flavor.
- For a spicier salad, add a pinch of crushed cayenne pepper flakes.

Storage tips

If not serving immediately, store the salad in an airtight container in the refrigerator for up to 2 days. It's best to enjoy the salad fresh to maintain the best quality and flavor.

Tips for allergens

- Ensure the olive oil is pure and not mixed with any other oils that might cause allergies.

Scientific references

- Research suggests that the high fiber content in zucchini and the monounsaturated fats in avocado can support liver and cardiovascular health, which contributes to lower cholesterol and improved liver function.

32. Beet and Carrot Liver Cleanse Juice

Beneficial effects

The Beet and Cucumber Liver Cleanse Juice is a potent detoxifier that supports liver health by aiding in the elimination of toxins and improving liver function. Beets are high in antioxidants and compounds that may help protect the liver from inflammation and oxidative stress. Cucumbers, replacing carrots, provide hydration and additional nutrients to enhance overall liver health. This juice also aids in digestion and boosts the immune system, making it a powerful addition to a liver-cleansing diet.

Portions	Preparation time
2 servings	10 minutes

Ingredients

- 2 medium beets, peeled and chopped
- 4 large cucumbers, peeled and chopped
- 1/2 lemon, peeled
- 1 inch piece of fresh ginger, peeled
- 1 cup of water

Instructions

1. Place the chopped beets, cucumbers, lemon, and ginger into a blender.
2. Add the water to help the ingredients blend smoothly.
3. Blend on high speed until the mixture is completely smooth.
4. Strain the juice through a fine mesh sieve or cheesecloth into a pitcher to remove the pulp, if desired.
5. Serve the juice immediately, or chill in the refrigerator for a refreshing cold drink.

Variations

- Add a handful of kale or dandelion greens for an extra nutrient boost without significantly altering the taste.
- For a sweeter juice, include an apple or a small amount of pure agave syrup.
- Incorporate a pinch of cayenne pepper for a spicy kick and additional detoxifying benefits.

Storage tips

This juice is best enjoyed fresh to maximize the benefits of its nutrients. However, if you need to store it, keep it in an airtight container in the refrigerator for up to 24 hours. Shake well before serving as separation may occur.

Tips for allergens

- For those with allergies to citrus, omit the lemon or replace it with a small amount of apple cider vinegar for a similar detoxifying effect.

- Ensure the water or coconut water used does not contain added flavors or preservatives that might cause allergic reactions.

PROMOTING HAIR GROWTH AND TREATING HAIR LOSS

Hair loss and thinning hair can be distressing, affecting not just our appearance but also our self-esteem. Fortunately, nature offers a bounty of remedies that can help nourish your scalp, strengthen your hair, and even promote new growth. Dr. Sebi's holistic approach emphasizes the importance of an alkaline diet, rich in minerals and vitamins, to support hair health from the inside out. Additionally, the use of specific herbs and natural treatments can provide external nourishment, creating the perfect environment for healthy hair growth.

First and foremost, an alkaline diet plays a crucial role in promoting hair growth and preventing hair loss. Foods rich in iron, zinc, and protein are essential for hair health. Leafy greens like lettuce and kale, along with nuts and seeds, are excellent sources of these nutrients. Alkaline water and herbal teas not only hydrate the body but also help in flushing out toxins that could be contributing to hair loss.

Incorporating specific herbs into your diet and hair care routine can also make a significant difference. For instance, horsetail, rich in silica, can strengthen hair strands, while rosemary has been shown to promote circulation in the scalp, encouraging hair growth. Nettle is another powerful herb that can combat hair loss, thanks to its high content of vitamins A and C, and minerals like iron and silica.

A simple yet effective hair care regimen can further support your efforts to promote hair growth and treat hair loss. Regular scalp massages with natural oils such as castor oil, which is known for its hair growth-promoting properties, or coconut oil, which moisturizes and repairs hair, can stimulate the hair follicles and enhance blood circulation to the scalp. This not only nourishes the hair roots but also helps in detoxifying the scalp, creating a healthy foundation for hair to grow.

Here's a step-by-step guide to creating a natural hair treatment oil that incorporates Dr. Sebi's principles:

Objective: To nourish the scalp and promote healthy hair growth using natural ingredients.

Preparation:

1. Gather all necessary materials and ingredients.

2. Ensure your workspace is clean to prevent any contamination of your natural hair treatment.

Materials:

- Castor oil (rich in fatty acids and known for promoting hair growth)

- Coconut oil (for its moisturizing properties)

- Rosemary essential oil (stimulates blood circulation in the scalp)

- Horsetail (optional, for its silica content)

Tools:

- Glass bowl

- Spoon for mixing

- Amber glass bottle for storage

Safety measures:

- Perform a patch test with the oils to ensure you're not allergic.

- Keep essential oils away from sensitive areas, such as the eyes.

Step-by-step instructions:

1. Start with 2 tablespoons of castor oil and 2 tablespoons of coconut oil as your base. Adjust the quantities based on the length and thickness of your hair.

2. If using, add a teaspoon of dried horsetail to the oils.

3. Warm the oils gently in a glass bowl. Do not microwave; use a double boiler method for safe heating.

4. Once the oils are warm (not hot), add 5-10 drops of rosemary essential oil. Stir well to combine.

5. Apply the oil mixture to your scalp with your fingertips, massaging gently in circular motions. Ensure the oil is distributed evenly throughout your scalp and hair.

6. Leave the treatment on for at least an hour or overnight for deep conditioning.

7. Wash your hair with a gentle, natural shampoo and condition as usual.

Cost estimate: Low to moderate, depending on the availability of ingredients.

Time estimate: Preparation time is about 10 minutes, with a minimum application time of 1 hour.

Safety tips:

- Ensure the oil mixture is at a comfortable temperature before applying to your scalp.

- Conduct a patch test before using essential oils to avoid allergic reactions.

Troubleshooting: If you find the oil mixture too heavy for your hair type, reduce the amount of castor oil and increase the coconut oil proportionately.

Maintenance: For best results, incorporate this treatment into your hair care routine once a week.

Difficulty rating: ★☆☆☆☆

Variations: You can substitute olive oil for coconut oil if you prefer or add other essential oils like lavender for additional benefits and fragrance.

By adopting Dr. Sebi's holistic approach to health, focusing on an alkaline diet, and using natural herbs and treatments, you can effectively promote hair growth and combat hair loss. Remember, consistency is key, and patience is crucial; natural remedies take time to show results. Embrace this journey towards healthier, stronger hair as part of your overall commitment to a healthier lifestyle.

Causes of Hair Loss

Hair loss, a concern that touches many, stems from a variety of causes, each influencing the scalp and hair's health in distinct ways. Understanding these causes is the first step towards addressing hair loss effectively and nurturing a healthier head of hair. One of the primary factors is genetics, playing a pivotal role in pattern baldness, which affects both men and women. This hereditary condition, known as androgenetic alopecia, is characterized by a gradual thinning of hair, leading to noticeable hair loss over time.

Hormonal changes and medical conditions also significantly contribute to hair loss. For instance, pregnancy, childbirth, menopause, and thyroid problems can all trigger hair shedding or thinning. Certain autoimmune diseases, such as alopecia areata, cause the body's immune system to attack hair follicles, resulting in patches of hair loss.

Nutritional deficiencies are another critical factor. A diet lacking in essential vitamins and minerals, such as iron, vitamin D, and zinc, can lead to weakened hair and increased hair fall. Protein is particularly vital for hair growth; thus, insufficient protein intake can also impact hair health negatively.

Stress, both physical and emotional, has a profound effect on hair growth cycles. High stress levels can push hair follicles into a resting phase, leading to increased hair shedding and noticeable thinning. This condition, known as telogen effluvium, is often temporary but can cause significant distress.

Certain hairstyles and treatments that pull on the hair, such as tight braids, ponytails, or chemical relaxers, can lead to a type of hair loss known as traction alopecia. Over time, these practices can damage hair follicles, leading to permanent hair loss if not addressed.

Environmental factors, including exposure to pollutants and UV radiation, can weaken hair and contribute to hair loss. Similarly, harsh hair care products and frequent use of heat styling tools can damage the hair shaft and follicles, leading to breakage and thinning.

Medications and medical treatments, such as chemotherapy, can have a significant impact on hair health. Some drugs, used to treat cancer, arthritis, depression, heart problems, and high blood pressure, can cause hair loss as a side effect. This type of hair loss is often temporary, but it can be distressing for those affected.

Infections of the scalp, such as ringworm, can also lead to hair loss. These conditions disrupt the normal functioning of hair follicles, causing patches of hair loss and, if left untreated, can lead to scarring and permanent hair loss.

By understanding the various causes of hair loss, individuals can take proactive steps towards addressing the underlying issues. Whether through dietary changes, stress management techniques, altering hair care practices, or seeking medical treatment for underlying conditions, there are many ways to combat hair loss and promote healthier hair growth. Remember, the key to effective hair loss treatment lies in identifying the cause and addressing it with a holistic approach that encompasses diet, lifestyle, and proper hair care practices.

Dr. Sebi's Herbal Remedies for Hair Health

Dr. Sebi's approach to hair health revolves around the principle that a clean, well-nourished body on the inside reflects on the outside, including the health of the hair. Emphasizing the importance of an alkaline diet, rich in vitamins, minerals, and hydration, is fundamental to supporting hair growth and strength. Additionally, Dr. Sebi advocated for the use of specific herbs and natural remedies to provide external nourishment and promote a healthy scalp, which is the foundation of healthy hair.

Key herbs identified by Dr. Sebi for supporting hair health include burdock root, which is known for its blood purifying properties and its ability to improve circulation to the scalp, thereby promoting hair growth.

Sarsaparilla, a lesser-known herb, is packed with antioxidants and vitamins that can help in strengthening hair and stimulating growth. Its anti-inflammatory properties also make it beneficial for those suffering from scalp conditions. Similarly, sea moss, rich in minerals and vitamins, nourishes the hair follicles and promotes a healthy, vibrant hair texture.

Incorporating these herbs into your hair care routine can be done through various methods, such as herbal rinses, oils, or masks. For instance, creating a herbal rinse with burdock root involves simmering the root in water to extract its beneficial properties, then cooling and straining the liquid. This rinse can be used after shampooing as a final rinse to stimulate the scalp and promote hair health.

For a nourishing hair oil, mix equal parts of aloe vera gel with coconut oil and add a few drops of rosemary essential oil. This combination can be massaged into the scalp and hair to moisturize, strengthen, and support growth. Leave the oil in your hair for at least an hour or overnight before washing out with a gentle shampoo.

A hair mask made from blended sea moss gel and a small amount of olive oil can be applied to the hair and scalp once a week. This mask will hydrate and provide essential nutrients directly to the follicles and scalp, encouraging healthier hair growth.

Remember, while external treatments are beneficial, the health of your hair is also a reflection of your overall health. Ensuring you are consuming an alkaline diet rich in fruits, vegetables, nuts, and seeds, staying hydrated, and managing stress are all crucial steps in promoting not only the health of your hair but your overall well-being.

Adopting Dr. Sebi's holistic approach to hair health encourages a return to natural, plant-based care, emphasizing the importance of internal health and the use of natural remedies to support hair growth and vitality. With patience and consistency, these practices can lead to stronger, healthier hair and a healthier you.

Nutritional Tips for Healthy Hair

Healthy hair starts from the inside out, and what you eat plays a pivotal role in hair health and growth. A balanced diet rich in specific nutrients can fortify hair strength, enhance growth, and combat hair loss. Key nutrients essential for healthy hair include proteins, vitamins, and minerals, each serving a unique function in maintaining hair health.

Proteins are the building blocks of hair, as hair is primarily made of keratin, a protein itself. Ensuring adequate protein intake through sources like garbanzo beans and legumes can help in the production and strengthening of hair strands. A lack of protein in the diet can lead to weak, brittle hair and, in severe cases, hair loss.

Vitamins play a crucial role in hair health, with Vitamin A, B-vitamins, Vitamin C, Vitamin D, and Vitamin E being particularly important. Vitamin A aids in the production of sebum, an oily substance secreted by the scalp, which keeps hair moisturized and healthy. B-vitamins, especially biotin, are renowned for their role in hair growth. Foods rich in B-vitamins include whole grains and dark, leafy greens. Vitamin C acts as an antioxidant and helps in the production of collagen, a protein that strengthens hair. Sources of Vitamin C include citrus fruits, strawberries, and bell peppers (except for green bell peppers). Vitamin D may also play a role in hair production, though research is ongoing. Mushrooms and fortified foods are good sources of Vitamin D, although in the case of the former, try to avoid shitake mushrooms. Vitamin E, another antioxidant, can help prevent oxidative stress, and is found in nuts, seeds, and green leafy vegetables.

Minerals such as iron, zinc, and selenium are also essential for hair health. Iron helps red blood cells carry oxygen to your cells, including hair follicles, and its deficiency can be associated with hair loss. Good sources of iron include red meat, chicken, fish, lentils, and iron-fortified cereals. Zinc plays a role in hair tissue growth and repair. It also helps keep the oil glands around the follicles working properly. Foods high in zinc include wheat germ and lentils. Selenium is an important mineral for the health of your hair and scalp, found in Brazil nuts and walnuts.

Hydration is another key aspect of maintaining healthy hair. Water is essential for transporting nutrients to the hair follicles. Without adequate hydration, hair can become dry, brittle, and more prone to breaking.

Incorporating a variety of these nutrient-rich foods into your diet can contribute significantly to the health and appearance of your hair. It's also important to note that while diet plays a crucial role in hair health, genetics, age, health conditions, and medications can also affect hair growth and health. If you're experiencing significant hair loss or other hair health issues, it's advisable to consult with a healthcare provider to determine the underlying cause and appropriate treatment.

By focusing on a nutrient-rich diet and ensuring you're getting a wide range of vitamins, minerals, and proteins, you can support your hair health from the inside out. Remember, changes in diet will take time to show in your hair, so patience and consistency with these nutritional habits are key.

Recipes for Treating Hair Loss

Harnessing the power of natural ingredients can be a transformative approach to treating hair loss. By focusing on recipes that incorporate the key nutrients previously discussed, you can create potent remedies that nourish the scalp and promote hair growth. Here are some effective recipes designed to combat hair loss and enhance the health of your hair.

33. Scalp Nourishing Hair Mask

Objective: To moisturize the scalp and strengthen hair follicles.

Preparation:
1. Gather all ingredients.
2. Mix in a bowl until a consistent paste is formed.

Materials:
- 1 ripe avocado (rich in vitamins B and E)
- 1 tablespoon of virgin coconut oil (moisturizes and promotes scalp health)
- 2 drops of rosemary essential oil (improves circulation)

Tools:
- Mixing bowl
- Fork or blender
- Application brush

Safety measures: Perform a patch test to ensure no allergic reactions to the ingredients.

Step-by-step instructions:
1. Mash the avocado in the mixing bowl until smooth.
2. Add the coconut oil to the avocado and mix thoroughly.
3. Incorporate the rosemary essential oil into the mixture.
4. Apply the mask to your scalp and hair, focusing on the roots.
5. Leave the mask on for 20-30 minutes.
6. Rinse off with lukewarm water and shampoo as usual.

Cost estimate: Low

Time estimate: 45 minutes

Safety tips: Ensure all ingredients are fresh and check for allergies.

Troubleshooting: If the mask is too thick, add a little water to adjust consistency.

Maintenance: Use once a week for best results.

Difficulty rating: ★☆☆☆☆

Variations: Substitute olive oil for coconut oil for additional moisture.

34. Stimulating Scalp Massage Oil

Objective: To stimulate hair growth by improving blood circulation to the scalp.

Preparation:
1. Measure and mix oils.
2. Store in a glass bottle.

Materials:
- 2 tablespoons of castor oil (rich in ricinoleic acid, promotes growth)
- 2 tablespoons of coconut oil (vitamins E and D, magnesium)
- 5 drops of peppermint essential oil (stimulates circulation)
- 5 drops of lavender essential oil (reduces stress and inflammation)

Tools:
- Measuring spoons
- Glass bottle for storage
- Dropper for application

Safety measures: Check for sensitivity to essential oils.

Step-by-step instructions:
1. Combine castor oil and coconut oil in the glass bottle.
2. Add the peppermint and lavender essential oils.
3. Close the bottle and shake well to mix.
4. Use the dropper to apply the oil directly to the scalp.
5. Massage gently in circular motions for 10-15 minutes.
6. Leave the oil in your hair for at least an hour or overnight for deep penetration.
7. Wash out with a gentle shampoo.

Cost estimate: Low

Time estimate: Overnight for best absorption

Safety tips: Conduct a patch test for the essential oils.

Troubleshooting: If irritation occurs, dilute the mixture with more carrier oil.

Maintenance: Apply 2-3 times a week for best results.

Difficulty rating: ★☆☆☆☆

Variations: Add vitamin E oil for an antioxidant boost.

35. Revitalizing Protein Hair Rinse

Objective: To provide protein to strengthen hair strands.

Preparation:
1. Brew herbal tea.
2. Add remaining ingredients and stir.

Materials:
- 1 cup of nettle tea (rich in silica and sulfur, promotes hair growth)
- 1 tablespoon of gelatin powder (a source of protein)
- 1 teaspoon of apple cider vinegar (restores pH balance)
- 2 drops of tea tree essential oil (cleanses the scalp)

Tools:
- Kettle or pot for brewing tea
- Measuring spoons
- Stirring spoon
- Container for mixture

Safety measures: Ensure the tea is not too hot before adding gelatin to prevent clumping.

Step-by-step instructions:
1. Brew a strong cup of nettle tea and let it cool slightly.
2. Dissolve the gelatin powder in the tea.
3. Add the apple cider vinegar and tea tree essential oil; stir well.
4. After shampooing, pour the rinse over your hair and scalp.
5. Leave it on for 5 minutes, then rinse with cool water.

Cost estimate: Low

Time estimate: 20 minutes

Safety tips: Use cool water for the final rinse to enhance shine and seal cuticles.

Troubleshooting: If the rinse leaves hair feeling sticky, reduce the amount of gelatin.

Maintenance: Use once a week to strengthen hair.

Difficulty rating: ★☆☆☆☆

Variations: Substitute chamomile tea for nettle tea for a soothing effect.

By incorporating these recipes into your hair care routine, you can address hair loss naturally and effectively. Remember, consistency is key to seeing results, and patience will guide you through your journey to healthier, stronger hair.

THE IMPORTANCE OF DETOXIFICATION

Detoxification plays a pivotal role in maintaining and restoring health, acting as a foundational element in Dr. Sebi's holistic approach to wellness. Our bodies are constantly bombarded with toxins from various sources, including processed foods, environmental pollutants, and stress, which can accumulate and impair our bodily functions. Detoxification is the process of removing these toxins, facilitating a return to optimal health and preventing disease.

The body naturally detoxifies itself through organs like the liver, kidneys, and skin. However, the overload of toxins in modern life can overwhelm these systems, leading to a buildup that can affect our health in numerous ways. Symptoms of toxin accumulation can include fatigue, headaches, digestive issues, skin problems, and more. By actively supporting the body's detoxification processes, we can help alleviate these symptoms and promote a state of vibrant health.

Dr. Sebi's detoxification methods emphasize the importance of an alkaline diet rich in whole, plant-based foods that naturally cleanse the body. Foods such as leafy greens, fruits, and herbs not only provide essential nutrients, but also support the body's natural detox pathways. For example, dandelion greens support liver function, a key organ in detoxification, while cucumbers and watermelons (avoid seedless, however) promote kidney health and hydration, aiding in the elimination of toxins.

In addition to dietary changes, Dr. Sebi recommends herbal teas and supplements that specifically target detoxification. Herbs like burdock root, sarsaparilla, and sea moss are integral to his protocols, each selected for their unique properties that support cleansing and healing. These herbs can be consumed as teas, tinctures, or capsules, offering a versatile approach to detoxification that can be tailored to individual needs.

Hydration is another critical aspect of detoxification. Drinking ample amounts of spring water not only helps to flush toxins from the body, but also supports overall cellular function. Hydration aids in the transport of nutrients to cells and the removal of waste products, a fundamental process in maintaining health.

Fasting or intermittent fasting is another method advocated by Dr. Sebi for detoxification. Periodic fasting gives the digestive system a rest, allowing the body to focus its energy on healing and eliminating toxins. During fasting, the consumption of herbal teas and alkaline water can enhance the detoxification process, providing the body with essential minerals and hydration.

Exercise and sweating are also beneficial for detoxification. Physical activity increases blood circulation and promotes the elimination of toxins through sweat. Incorporating gentle exercises such as walking, yoga, or rebounding can support the body's natural detox pathways while contributing to overall physical and mental well-being.

Implementing these detoxification strategies can lead to significant improvements in health, including increased energy, clearer skin, improved digestion, and a greater sense of overall well-being. It's important to approach detoxification as a gentle, ongoing process rather than a one-time event. Making consistent, healthful choices supports the body's natural ability to cleanse and heal, aligning with Dr. Sebi's philosophy of living in harmony with nature for optimal health.

By embracing detoxification as a key component of a holistic health regimen, individuals can take proactive steps towards preventing disease and achieving a state of vibrant health. Dr. Sebi's teachings provide a blueprint for detoxification that is accessible, effective, and grounded in the wisdom of natural healing.

The Role of Detoxification in Health

Detoxification is a natural and critical process that our bodies perform to maintain health and vitality. It involves the elimination of toxins from the body, which can come from various sources including the food we eat, the air we breathe, and the products we use. Toxins can accumulate in our bodies over time, leading to a variety of health issues such as fatigue, headaches, weight gain, and more serious chronic diseases. The role of detoxification in health is to support the body's natural ability to cleanse itself, ensuring that these toxins are efficiently removed and that our organs function optimally.

The liver, kidneys, intestines, lungs, lymphatic system, and skin all play a part in the detoxification process. Each organ works to filter out toxins from the blood, break them down, and eliminate them through urine, feces, sweat, and exhalation. For instance, the liver filters toxins and processes them for safe removal, while the kidneys filter our blood and remove waste through urine. However, when these systems are overwhelmed by excessive toxins, their efficiency can be compromised, leading to an accumulation of waste products in our bodies.

An effective way to support the body's detoxification process is through diet. Consuming a diet rich in whole, plant-based foods that are high in nutrients and antioxidants can help to enhance the body's natural detox mechanisms. Foods such as leafy greens, berries, garlic, and beets are known for their detoxifying properties. These foods provide the body with the necessary vitamins, minerals, and antioxidants that support liver function and help in the elimination of toxins.

Herbal teas and supplements can also play a significant role in supporting detoxification. Herbs such as milk thistle, dandelion root, and burdock are known for their liver-supporting properties. They can help to stimulate bile production, which assists in the digestion of fats and the elimination of toxins from the body. Drinking herbal teas or taking supplements containing these herbs can be an effective way to enhance the body's detoxification processes.

Hydration is another key factor in detoxification. Water is essential for the proper functioning of every cell in the body and helps to flush toxins out through the kidneys. Drinking adequate amounts of clean, filtered water each day can help to ensure that toxins are efficiently removed from the body.

Physical activity and sweating are also beneficial for detoxification. Exercise increases blood circulation, which helps to transport nutrients to our cells and waste products away from them. Sweating, a natural detoxification process, helps to eliminate toxins through the skin. Engaging in regular physical activity, such as walking, yoga, or cycling, can support the body's natural detox pathways.

Incorporating fasting or intermittent fasting into one's routine can give the digestive system a rest and allow the body to focus on detoxification and healing. During periods of fasting, the body has the opportunity to repair and regenerate its cells, which can enhance the detoxification process.

In summary, detoxification is an essential process for maintaining health and preventing disease. By supporting the body's natural detox pathways through diet, hydration, herbal supplements, physical activity, and fasting, individuals can help to ensure that toxins are efficiently removed from the body. This can lead to improved energy levels, better digestion, clearer skin, and overall better health. Embracing a lifestyle that supports detoxification aligns with Dr. Sebi's philosophy of living in harmony with nature and utilizing natural methods to achieve optimal health.

Dr. Sebi's Detoxification Methods Explained

Dr. Sebi's detoxification methods are grounded in the principle that a clean body is the foundation for optimal health. His approach is holistic, focusing on cleansing the body from the inside out to prevent disease, restore health, and maintain vitality. Central to his methodology is the belief that removing accumulated toxins and waste products from the body can significantly improve physical and mental well-being. Dr. Sebi's detoxification strategies are designed to support the body's natural detox pathways, emphasizing the importance of an alkaline diet, herbal teas, fasting, hydration, and physical activity.

An alkaline diet plays a crucial role in Dr. Sebi's detoxification process. This diet includes a high intake of whole, plant-based foods such as fruits, vegetables, nuts, seeds, and alkaline grains. These foods are selected for their mineral content, hydration properties, and their ability to alkalize the body, creating an environment that discourages disease. By focusing on nutrient-dense, minimally processed foods, this diet aids in the elimination of toxins and supports the body's natural healing processes.

Herbal teas are another cornerstone of Dr. Sebi's detox methods. Herbs like burdock root, sarsaparilla, and sea moss are celebrated for their detoxifying properties. These herbs support various organs and systems in the body, including the liver, kidneys, and lymphatic system, which are critical for removing toxins. Consuming these herbal teas regularly can help cleanse the blood, improve organ function, and enhance overall health.

Fasting, according to Dr. Sebi, is a powerful detoxification tool. By temporarily abstaining from food, the body is given a break from digestion, which allows it to focus its energy on healing and detoxification. During fasting periods, the consumption of herbal teas and alkaline water is encouraged to support the body's cleansing processes, providing essential minerals and aiding in hydration.

Hydration is essential for effective detoxification. Dr. Sebi emphasizes the importance of drinking plenty of spring water to help flush toxins from the body. Adequate hydration supports kidney function, aids in digestion, and ensures that cells are nourished and waste products are efficiently removed. Water is not just a transporter of nutrients and waste, but also vital for maintaining cellular health and integrity.

Physical activity and sweating are natural detoxification methods that complement Dr. Sebi's dietary recommendations. Exercise increases blood circulation, which enhances the delivery of nutrients to cells and the removal of waste products. Sweating, a direct result of physical activity, is one of the body's primary methods of eliminating toxins. Incorporating gentle, regular exercise into one's routine, such as walking, yoga, or rebounding, can significantly support the body's detox pathways.

By integrating these detoxification methods into daily life, individuals can take proactive steps toward improving their health. Dr. Sebi's approach is not about quick fixes but rather about making sustainable lifestyle changes that honor the body's natural ability to heal itself. Embracing these practices can lead to increased energy, clearer skin, improved digestion, and a greater sense of well-being. It's a journey of transformation that aligns with the natural rhythms of the body and the healing power of nature.

Step-by-Step Detox Plans

Embarking on a detox plan can rejuvenate your body, mind, and spirit, aligning with Dr. Sebi's principles of natural healing and wellness. Here, we outline a simple yet effective step-by-step detox plan that can be easily incorporated into your daily routine. This plan focuses on leveraging the power of alkaline foods, herbal teas, hydration, and physical activity to support your body's natural detoxification processes.

Objective: To cleanse the body of toxins and support overall health through natural methods.

Preparation:

1. Plan your detox period. A 3 to 7-day window is ideal for beginners.

2. Clear your schedule as much as possible to allow for rest and relaxation.

3. Shop for necessary ingredients and supplies ahead of time.

Materials:

- Alkaline foods (leafy greens, fruits, nuts, seeds, and alkaline grains)
- Herbal teas (dandelion, burdock root, sarsaparilla)
- Spring water
- Fresh herbs and spices

Tools:

- Blender for smoothies
- Tea kettle or pot for brewing herbal teas
- Water bottle to ensure hydration throughout the day

Safety measures:

- Consult with a healthcare provider before starting if you have any health conditions or concerns.
- Ensure all herbs and supplements are safe for consumption and do not interfere with any medications you are taking.

Step-by-step instructions:

1. Morning Ritual: Start each day with a glass of warm spring water with lemon to stimulate digestion and liver function.

2. Breakfast: Consume a smoothie made with alkaline fruits, leafy greens, and a tablespoon of sea moss gel for minerals and hydration.

3. Mid-Morning: Sip on dandelion herbal tea to support liver detoxification. Stay hydrated with spring water throughout the morning.

4. Lunch: Prepare a salad with a variety of leafy greens, sprouts, cucumber, avocado, and a dressing made from lime juice and cold-pressed olive oil. This meal is rich in fiber and alkaline to support detoxification.

5. Afternoon Snack: Enjoy a piece of alkaline fruit, such as an apple or a few slices of watermelon (but not seedless), to keep energy levels up and support kidney detoxification.

6. Dinner: Make a light vegetable soup with alkaline vegetables and herbs. Include ingredients like kale, onions, and seaweed for their detoxifying properties.

7. **Evening Ritual:** Drink a cup of burdock root or sarsaparilla tea to further support the cleansing of the blood and organs.

8. **Throughout the Day:** Ensure you drink plenty of spring water, aiming for at least 8 glasses to facilitate toxin elimination through urine.

9. **Physical Activity:** Engage in gentle exercise daily, such as walking, yoga, or stretching, to promote circulation and toxin elimination through sweat.

10. **Rest and Reflect:** Dedicate at least 7-8 hours each night for restful sleep. Use this detox period for introspection or meditation to support mental and emotional detoxification.

Cost estimate: Low to moderate, depending on the availability of fresh produce and herbs.

Time estimate: 3 to 7 days, based on personal preference and response to the detox.

Safety tips:

- Listen to your body. If you feel excessively tired or unwell, adjust the detox plan accordingly.

- Stay hydrated to help facilitate the detox process and avoid dehydration.

Troubleshooting:

- If you experience headaches or dizziness, ensure you are adequately hydrated and not fasting too aggressively. Adjust your intake of solid foods as needed.

Maintenance: After completing the detox plan, gradually reintroduce other foods into your diet, focusing on maintaining a high intake of whole, plant-based foods and minimizing processed foods and sugars.

Difficulty rating: ★★☆☆☆ - This detox plan is designed to be accessible for beginners, with a focus on simplicity and ease of implementation.

Variations: Customize the plan by incorporating different alkaline foods and herbal teas based on availability and personal preference. The key is to maintain an emphasis on natural, whole foods and hydration to support the body's detoxification processes.

By following this step-by-step detox plan, you can support your body's natural ability to cleanse and rejuvenate, paving the way for improved health and vitality in alignment with Dr. Sebi's holistic approach to wellness.

DR. SEBI'S RECOMMENDED LIFESTYLE CHANGES

Adopting Dr. Sebi's recommended lifestyle changes is a transformative journey towards achieving optimal health and well-being, focusing on natural healing and the power of an alkaline diet. Embracing these changes requires a holistic approach, considering not just what we eat but how we live. Dr. Sebi's guidance encourages us to align our daily habits with the principles of natural living, ensuring that our bodies function at their best.

First and foremost, stress management plays a crucial role in maintaining health. In today's fast-paced world, stress is a common ailment that can lead to a host of health issues, including high blood pressure, heart disease, and weakened immune function. Dr. Sebi emphasized the importance of incorporating practices such as meditation, deep breathing exercises, and spending time in nature to reduce stress levels. These practices not only calm the mind, but also enhance our connection to the earth, grounding us in the present moment.

Exercise is another pillar of Dr. Sebi's lifestyle recommendations. Regular physical activity is essential for overall health, improving cardiovascular function, boosting mood, and enhancing energy levels. Dr. Sebi advocated for gentle, natural forms of exercise such as walking, yoga, and swimming. These activities promote blood circulation and help in the detoxification process by encouraging sweating, a natural way for the body to eliminate toxins.

Sleep and recovery are equally important in Dr. Sebi's holistic health approach. Adequate rest is crucial for the body to heal, regenerate, and detoxify. Dr. Sebi recommended creating a peaceful bedtime routine to ensure restful sleep, including turning off electronic devices an hour before bed, sleeping in a dark, cool room, and aiming for 7-9 hours of sleep each night. Restorative sleep supports the body's natural rhythms and healing processes, allowing us to wake up refreshed and energized.

Avoiding environmental toxins is another key aspect of Dr. Sebi's lifestyle changes. In our modern world, we are exposed to a myriad of chemicals and pollutants that can be harmful to our health. Dr. Sebi advised being mindful of the products we use on our bodies and in our homes, opting for natural, organic options whenever possible. This includes personal care products, cleaning supplies, and even the water we drink. By reducing our exposure to harmful chemicals, we support our body's natural ability to detoxify and maintain health.

Incorporating these lifestyle changes into our daily routines can have a profound impact on our health and well-being. Dr. Sebi's teachings encourage us to live in harmony with nature, making choices that support our body's natural healing abilities. By managing stress, engaging in regular physical activity, prioritizing restful sleep, and minimizing exposure to toxins, we can create a foundation for lasting health and vitality. These changes, coupled with an alkaline diet rich in natural, plant-based foods, offer a powerful pathway to healing and wellness, embodying Dr. Sebi's vision of a life lived in balance and harmony with the natural world.

Stress Management and Mental Health

Managing stress and nurturing mental health are essential components of a holistic approach to wellness. In a world where stressors abound, finding effective ways to cope and maintain a balanced mental state is crucial. Dr. Sebi's teachings emphasize the interconnectedness of body and mind, advocating for natural methods to support both physical and mental well-being. By adopting practices that reduce stress and enhance mental health, individuals can achieve a greater sense of harmony and vitality.

Meditation is a powerful tool for stress management. It involves sitting quietly and focusing on the breath, a mantra, or a specific thought to calm the mind. Regular meditation practice can significantly lower stress levels, reduce anxiety, and improve mood. It's a practice that requires no special equipment or environment and can be done anywhere, making it accessible to everyone. Starting with just a few minutes a day and gradually increasing the time can make meditation a manageable and beneficial part of your daily routine.

Deep breathing exercises are another simple yet effective technique for managing stress. Deep, diaphragmatic breathing helps activate the body's relaxation response, counteracting the effects of stress. Techniques such as the 4-7-8 method, where you inhale deeply for 4 seconds, hold the breath for 7 seconds, and exhale slowly for 8 seconds, can be particularly helpful. Incorporating these exercises into your daily life, especially during moments of heightened stress, can provide immediate relief and promote a sense of calm.

Spending time in nature has been shown to have a profound impact on mental health. Nature's tranquility can help reduce stress, improve mood, and enhance cognitive function. Whether it's a walk in the park, gardening, or simply sitting outside and appreciating the natural surroundings, connecting with nature is a therapeutic practice that supports mental well-being. Encouraging regular outdoor activities can be a simple yet effective way to combat stress and nurture a positive mental state.

Physical activity is not only beneficial for physical health, but also for mental health. Exercise releases endorphins, chemicals in the brain that act as natural painkillers and mood elevators. Engaging in regular physical activity, such as walking, yoga, or any form of exercise that you enjoy, can help reduce stress, alleviate symptoms of depression and anxiety, and boost overall mood. Finding an activity that you look forward to can make exercise an enjoyable and sustainable part of your lifestyle.

A balanced diet plays a significant role in mental health. Consuming a diet rich in whole, plant-based foods provides the body with essential nutrients that support brain function and mood regulation. Foods high in antioxidants, omega-3 fatty acids, and vitamins can help combat stress and promote mental well-being. Incorporating alkaline foods, as recommended by Dr. Sebi, can further enhance this effect, supporting both physical and mental health.

Building a support system of family, friends, or a community that shares similar health and wellness goals can provide emotional support and encouragement. Sharing experiences, challenges, and successes with others can help reduce feelings of isolation, increase motivation, and foster a sense of belonging. Engaging in group activities, whether related to exercise, meditation, or simply social gatherings, can enhance mental health and provide a valuable outlet for stress relief.

By integrating these practices into daily life, individuals can effectively manage stress and support their mental health. Embracing a holistic approach to wellness, as advocated by Dr. Sebi, involves nurturing both the body and the mind. Through meditation, deep breathing, connecting with nature, physical activity, a balanced diet, and building a supportive community, individuals can achieve a greater sense of peace, balance, and well-being.

Importance of Exercise

Exercise is a cornerstone of maintaining a healthy lifestyle, and its benefits extend far beyond weight management. Engaging in regular physical activity is crucial for enhancing cardiovascular health, improving muscle strength, boosting mental health, and supporting the body's detoxification processes. For individuals embarking on a journey toward natural healing and wellness, incorporating exercise into daily routines can significantly amplify the effects of dietary changes and other lifestyle adjustments recommended by Dr. Sebi.

Cardiovascular health is directly impacted by exercise. Regular physical activity helps to strengthen the heart, allowing it to pump blood more efficiently throughout the body. This not only reduces the risk of heart disease but also lowers blood pressure and improves cholesterol levels. Simple activities such as brisk walking, cycling, or swimming for at least 30 minutes a day can make a substantial difference in heart health.

Muscle strength and endurance are also enhanced through exercise. Engaging in strength training or resistance exercises a few times a week can help build muscle mass, which is essential for metabolism and overall physical stability. Strong muscles contribute to better posture, reduce the risk of injuries, and improve the ability to perform daily tasks with ease.

The mental health benefits of exercise are profound. Physical activity releases endorphins, often referred to as feel-good hormones, which can alleviate feelings of stress, depression, and anxiety. Exercise also promotes better sleep patterns, which is crucial for mental and emotional well-being. Activities such as yoga and tai chi, in addition to providing physical benefits, offer a meditative experience that can help calm the mind and reduce stress.

Exercise plays a vital role in the body's detoxification process. By promoting sweating, it helps to eliminate toxins through the skin. Additionally, increased circulation during exercise enhances the delivery of oxygen and nutrients to tissues while facilitating the removal of waste products. Engaging in regular physical activity supports the function of the lymphatic system, which plays a key role in immune health and detoxification.

For those new to exercise, starting with gentle activities and gradually increasing intensity is key to building a sustainable routine. Listening to the body and incorporating a variety of exercises can prevent boredom and reduce the risk of injury. It's important to find activities that are enjoyable, whether it's dancing, hiking, or participating in team sports, as this will encourage consistency and long-term commitment.

Hydration is essential when exercising, especially during activities that promote sweating. Drinking plenty of water before, during, and after exercise supports hydration and aids in the detoxification process. Additionally, wearing appropriate clothing and footwear can enhance comfort and performance while minimizing the risk of injury.

Incorporating exercise into daily life is a powerful way to enhance the body's natural healing abilities and support overall health and wellness. By making physical activity a regular part of the routine, individuals can enjoy the numerous benefits that exercise offers, aligning with Dr. Sebi's holistic approach to health and living in harmony with nature.

Sleep and Recovery

Adequate sleep and proper recovery are foundational elements in the holistic approach to health and well-being, aligning perfectly with Dr. Sebi's teachings on natural healing. The body uses sleep to repair muscles, consolidate memories, and regulate hormones that control appetite and growth—making it a critical component of overall health. Without sufficient sleep, the body cannot fully benefit from the nutrients and herbs that are part of Dr. Sebi's dietary recommendations, nor can it effectively detoxify and heal.

The quality of sleep directly impacts the body's ability to recover from daily stressors, both physical and mental. During deep sleep stages, the body releases growth hormones that aid in cell regeneration and repair. This process is crucial for maintaining a strong immune system, supporting cardiovascular health, and managing stress. Furthermore, sleep plays a vital role in cognitive function, affecting concentration, decision-making, and mood. Chronic sleep deprivation can lead to a host of health issues, including obesity, diabetes, cardiovascular disease, and depression.

Creating a conducive sleep environment is key to enhancing sleep quality. This involves maintaining a cool, dark, and quiet bedroom. Investing in a comfortable mattress and pillows can also significantly improve sleep quality. The use of electronic devices should be minimized before bedtime, as the blue light emitted by screens can interfere with the body's natural circadian rhythms, making it harder to fall asleep.

Establishing a consistent sleep schedule further supports the body's internal clock, signaling to the body when it's time to wind down and prepare for sleep. Going to bed and waking up at the same time each day, even on weekends, can help stabilize sleep patterns and improve the quality of sleep.

Incorporating relaxation techniques into the evening routine can also aid in falling asleep more easily. Practices such as reading, taking a warm bath, or engaging in gentle yoga or meditation can help calm the mind and prepare the body for rest. Herbal teas, such as chamomile or valerian root, are known for their natural sedative properties and can be a beneficial part of a nighttime routine.

Diet plays a significant role in sleep quality as well. Consuming alkaline foods that are rich in magnesium and potassium, such as bananas, avocados, and leafy greens, can help relax the muscles and nervous system, promoting better sleep. It's also important to avoid heavy meals, caffeine, and sugar close to bedtime, as these can disrupt sleep.

Physical activity during the day can enhance sleep at night. Regular exercise, particularly in the morning or afternoon, can help deepen sleep. However, intense workouts should be avoided in the hours leading up to bedtime, as they can increase energy levels and make it more difficult to fall asleep.

For those struggling with sleep issues, it's crucial to address any underlying conditions that may be contributing to the problem. Consulting with a healthcare provider can help identify and treat sleep disorders such as insomnia, sleep apnea, or restless leg syndrome.

In summary, sleep and recovery are integral to the body's ability to heal and thrive. By prioritizing sleep and creating habits that support restful nights, individuals can enhance their physical, mental, and emotional health, embodying the principles of Dr. Sebi's holistic approach to wellness.

Avoiding Environmental Toxins

Living in today's world, we're surrounded by environmental toxins at every turn, from the air we breathe to the food we eat and even the products we use daily. These toxins can have a profound impact on our health, contributing to chronic diseases, disrupting our hormonal balance, and weakening our immune system. But fear not, there are practical steps we can take to minimize our exposure and protect our health, aligning perfectly with Dr. Sebi's teachings on living in harmony with nature.

First off, let's talk about the air we breathe. Air pollution, both indoor and outdoor, is a significant source of environmental toxins. Investing in a high-quality air purifier can help remove pollutants from your indoor environment, making your home a safer haven. Additionally, incorporating indoor plants like spider plants, peace lilies, and snake plants can naturally purify the air, as they absorb toxins and produce oxygen.

When it comes to the food we eat, opting for organic produce whenever possible is a key step in avoiding pesticides and genetically modified organisms (GMOs) that can disrupt our body's natural functions. Washing fruits and vegetables with a mixture of baking soda and water can help remove some of the surface pesticides if organic options aren't accessible. Moreover, reducing the consumption of processed foods, which often contain harmful additives and preservatives, supports our body's natural detoxification processes.

Personal care and household cleaning products are also major sources of everyday toxins. Switching to natural, non-toxic products for cleaning, laundry, and personal care can significantly reduce your exposure. Look for products with simple, recognizable ingredients or consider making your own. Common household items like vinegar, baking soda, and lemon can be powerful natural cleaners, while coconut oil, shea butter, and essential oils can be used to create effective personal care products.

Water is the essence of life, yet it can also be a source of toxins due to contamination with chemicals like chlorine and heavy metals. Investing in a good quality water filter for your home can ensure that you're drinking and cooking with clean water, further reducing your toxin load. Remember, hydration plays a crucial role in detoxification, helping to flush toxins out of your body.

Lastly, minimizing electronic pollution is something many of us overlook. Electromagnetic fields (EMFs) from cell phones, computers, and Wi-Fi routers can impact our health over time. Reducing exposure by turning off electronic devices when not in use, keeping cell phones away from the body, and even considering wired internet connections can help mitigate these effects.

By taking these steps to avoid environmental toxins, we're not only protecting our health but also supporting the body's natural ability to heal and maintain balance, as Dr. Sebi emphasized. Remember, every small change we make contributes to a larger impact on our well-being and the planet.

PRACTICAL TIPS AND TRICKS FOR DAILY LIFE

Maintaining a balanced pH level in your daily life is simpler than it might seem at first glance. The key is incorporating alkaline foods into your diet, which can naturally help your body maintain its optimal pH balance. Start by adding more leafy greens, cucumbers, avocados, and alkaline water to your meals. These foods are not only packed with nutrients but also have alkalizing effects on the body, helping to counteract the acidity that can come from processed foods and environmental toxins.

When it comes to hydration, remember that not all water is created equal. Alkaline water, which has a higher pH level than regular tap water, can be a beneficial addition to your diet. It helps to neutralize acid in the bloodstream, leading to increased oxygen levels and improved energy and metabolism. If alkaline water isn't readily available, consider adding a squeeze of lemon or lime to your water. Despite their acidic taste, these fruits create an alkalizing effect once metabolized.

Reading food labels is another practical tip that can have a significant impact on your health. It's important to be aware of the ingredients in the foods you consume. Look for foods with short, recognizable ingredient lists, and avoid those with artificial additives, preservatives, and high levels of sugar and salt. Opting for whole, unprocessed foods whenever possible is a simple way to ensure you're nourishing your body with the best nutrients available.

Building a support system can also play a crucial role in maintaining a healthy lifestyle. Surrounding yourself with like-minded individuals who share your health and wellness goals can provide motivation, accountability, and encouragement. Whether it's joining a local fitness class, participating in an online health forum, or simply sharing recipes and tips with friends, having a community can make all the difference in staying on track with your health journey.

Here are 5 easy and healthy recipes to get you started on incorporating more alkaline foods into your diet:

1. Alkaline Morning Smoothie: Blend kale, cucumber, green apple, and a slice of ginger with coconut water for a refreshing and energizing start to your day.

2. Quinoa and Avocado Salad: Mix cooked quinoa with diced avocado, cherry tomatoes, cucumber, and a dressing of lemon juice, olive oil, salt for a quick and nutritious lunch.

3. Stuffed Bell Peppers: Fill halved bell peppers with a mixture of sautéed mushrooms, quinoa, and spices, then bake until tender. A perfect alkaline dinner option.

4. Alkaline Snack Bars: Combine almond butter, dried coconut, and agave syrup. Press into a pan, chill, and then cut into bars for a healthy snack on the go.

5. Herbal Alkaline Tea: Steep fresh mint, fennel, and lemon balm in hot water for a soothing and alkalizing herbal tea.

By incorporating these practical tips and tricks into your daily life, you can take significant steps toward improving your well-being and aligning with Dr. Sebi's principles of natural health. Remember, the journey to better health is a marathon, not a sprint. Small, consistent changes can lead to lasting benefits over time.

Maintaining a Balanced pH Level

Maintaining a balanced pH level in the body is crucial for optimal health and well-being. The pH scale, which ranges from 0 to 14, measures how acidic or alkaline a substance is. A pH of 7 is considered neutral, below 7 acidic, and above 7 alkaline. The human body thrives in a slightly alkaline environment, with an ideal blood pH level of around 7.4. When the body's pH level is balanced, cells function properly, and the body can effectively fight off diseases. However, an overly acidic environment can lead to a host of health issues, including inflammation, decreased immunity, and diseases such as arthritis and cancer.

The modern diet, rich in processed foods, meat, dairy, and sugar, tends to be highly acidic. This, combined with stress and environmental toxins, can push our body's pH balance towards acidity. To counteract this, incorporating more alkaline foods into your diet is essential. Alkaline foods help neutralize the body's acidity, support detoxification, and promote healing.

Focus on eating plenty of leafy greens, vegetables, fruits, nuts, seeds, and whole grains. These foods not only support a balanced pH but also provide vital nutrients and antioxidants that promote health.

Hydration is another key factor in maintaining a balanced pH level. Drinking plenty of water helps flush toxins from the body and keeps the system functioning optimally. Aim for at least 8 glasses of water a day, and consider adding lemon or lime to your water. Despite their initial acidity, these fruits become alkaline in the body and can help raise your pH level.

Exercise also plays a role in maintaining pH balance. Regular physical activity helps release acids from the body through sweat. Additionally, exercise boosts circulation and oxygenation of the body's cells, supporting overall health and helping to maintain an alkaline environment.

Stress management is equally important. Chronic stress can lead to acid buildup in the body, so finding ways to relax and de-stress is crucial. Practices such as yoga, meditation, deep breathing, and spending time in nature can help reduce stress levels and support a balanced pH.

Finally, monitoring your pH level can provide valuable insights into your body's state of balance. pH test strips are available at most health food stores and can be used to test your saliva or urine. While these tests are not as accurate as blood tests, they can give you a general idea of your body's pH level and help you make adjustments to your diet and lifestyle as needed.

By focusing on alkaline foods, staying hydrated, exercising regularly, managing stress, and monitoring your pH levels, you can help ensure your body maintains its optimal pH balance. This, in turn, supports your overall health and well-being, allowing you to lead a vibrant, energetic life. Remember, small, consistent changes can have a profound impact on your health, so start incorporating these practices into your daily routine today.

Reading Food Labels

Reading food labels is a crucial skill for anyone looking to maintain a healthy and balanced diet, especially when following Dr. Sebi's principles of natural healing and alkaline eating. Food labels provide essential information about the nutritional content of food items, helping you make informed choices about what you're putting into your body. To start, focus on the serving size and servings per container, which can be surprisingly revealing. Many products might seem healthy at a glance, but a closer look at the serving size might show that you're consuming more calories, sugar, or sodium than you intended.

Next, pay attention to the list of ingredients. Ingredients are listed in order of quantity, from highest to lowest. This means the first few ingredients make up the bulk of the product. Dr. Sebi's teachings emphasize the importance of consuming natural, whole foods, so be wary of long lists of ingredients, especially those that are difficult to pronounce or sound like chemical compounds. These are often artificial additives, preservatives, and flavorings that are best avoided. Instead, look for foods with simple, whole-food ingredients, ideally ones that you could find and use in your own kitchen.

The nutritional facts panel is another key area to focus on. Here, you'll find information on calories, fats, cholesterol, sodium, carbohydrates, fiber, sugars, and protein. Dr. Sebi's alkaline diet encourages the consumption of foods that are low in sodium and high in minerals and vitamins. Therefore, aim for foods that are low in sodium and have no added sugars. High fiber content is also a plus, as it supports digestive health and can help maintain a feeling of fullness, reducing the likelihood of overeating.

Another important aspect to consider is the presence of vitamins and minerals. Dr. Sebi highlighted the importance of consuming mineral-rich foods to support the body's healing and maintenance. Look for foods that are high in essential vitamins and minerals, such as vitamin C, iron, calcium, and magnesium. These nutrients play a crucial role in supporting overall health and well-being, aligning with the natural healing approach.

Lastly, be mindful of health claims on packaging. Phrases like "all-natural," "low-fat," or "supports immunity" can be misleading. These claims are not always backed by substantial evidence and can be used as marketing tactics to make products appear healthier than they actually are. Instead of relying solely on these claims, use the information on the food label to make your own assessment of the product's nutritional value.

Incorporating these tips into your daily routine can empower you to make healthier food choices that align with Dr. Sebi's teachings. By understanding how to read food labels effectively, you can avoid processed and artificial foods, opting instead for natural, nutrient-rich foods that support your body's health and vitality. Remember, the goal is to nourish your body with high-quality, alkaline foods that promote healing and well-being, and becoming proficient in reading food labels is a significant step in that direction.

Building a Support System

Building a support system is a fundamental step in maintaining and enhancing your journey toward a healthier lifestyle, especially when adopting the principles of Dr. Sebi's alkaline diet and holistic health approach. A strong support system can provide encouragement, share knowledge, and offer motivation, making it easier to navigate challenges and celebrate successes. It's about creating a network of friends, family, and community members who understand and respect your health and wellness goals, providing a sense of belonging and accountability that can be incredibly empowering.

To start building this support system, first, identify individuals in your life who are open-minded, supportive, or perhaps even on their own health journey. These could be friends interested in natural health, family members who have shown support for your choices, or colleagues who share similar wellness goals. Engaging with these people about your health objectives, sharing what you've learned, and discussing the benefits of a natural, alkaline lifestyle can help foster a supportive environment.

Joining local or online communities focused on holistic health, natural healing, and the alkaline diet can also expand your support network. Many cities have groups that meet regularly to share experiences, recipes, and tips. Online forums, social media groups, and health blogs can connect you with a broader community of like-minded individuals from around the world. Participating in these communities not only offers support but also provides a wealth of knowledge and resources that can aid in your health journey.

Another key aspect of building a support system is finding a mentor or coach, someone who has experience and knowledge in the areas you're exploring. This could be a holistic health practitioner, a nutritionist familiar with the alkaline diet, or someone who has successfully incorporated Dr. Sebi's principles into their life. A mentor can offer personalized advice, help you navigate obstacles, and provide encouragement based on their own experiences.

It's also important to communicate your goals and needs clearly with those around you. Sharing why you're making these lifestyle changes and explaining the benefits can help others understand your choices and how they can support you. Whether it's asking family members to consider trying new recipes at home, inviting friends to join you for nature walks, or simply requesting their encouragement, clear communication is key to building and maintaining a supportive environment.

Lastly, remember to be a support system for others as well. Sharing your journey, the challenges you've faced, and the successes you've achieved can inspire and motivate those around you. Offering your support, listening to others' experiences, and celebrating their achievements can strengthen your relationships and foster a mutually supportive community.

Building a support system is an ongoing process that evolves as you continue on your health journey. By surrounding yourself with positive influences, seeking out knowledge and encouragement, and offering the same in return, you can create a powerful network that supports your goals of living a healthier, more balanced life. This community not only enriches your journey but also contributes to a larger movement toward holistic health and wellness.

CONCLUSION

Embarking on a journey toward better health through Dr. Sebi's teachings, you've explored the transformative power of natural healing, the alkaline diet, and the importance of detoxification. Embracing these principles offers a path to address various health challenges holistically, focusing on the body's innate ability to heal itself when supported with the right nutrients and environment. The journey doesn't end here; it's an ongoing process of learning, experimenting, and adapting to what best supports your body and well-being. Remember, small, consistent steps can lead to significant changes, empowering you to take control of your health and live in harmony with nature. As you continue to incorporate these teachings into your daily life, stay curious, open-minded, and supportive of yourself and others seeking a similar path. Your health journey is uniquely yours, but it's also part of a larger collective seeking to reclaim well-being through natural, holistic means.

Recap of Key Points

Throughout this book, we've journeyed through Dr. Sebi's holistic approach to health, emphasizing the power of the alkaline diet, the significance of detoxification, and the use of natural herbs for healing. Dr. Sebi's methodology, grounded in the belief that a properly nourished body can heal itself, advocates for a diet rich in alkaline foods to maintain the body's pH balance, thereby promoting overall well-being and preventing disease. Key to this approach is the consumption of whole, plant-based foods and the avoidance of acidic, processed foods, which can disrupt the body's natural state and lead to health issues.

We've explored specific dietary recommendations and herbal remedies for a range of conditions, from herpes and HIV to diabetes, high blood pressure, lupus, kidney diseases, and cancer, underscoring the importance of supporting the body's immune system and detoxification processes. Recipes tailored to each condition offer practical, delicious ways to incorporate these principles into daily life, making it easier to adopt a healthier lifestyle.

Detoxification, a cornerstone of Dr. Sebi's teachings, has been highlighted as a vital process for removing toxins from the body, with specific detox plans and herbal teas designed to support liver, kidney, and lymphatic health. The book also delves into lifestyle changes recommended by Dr. Sebi, including stress management, exercise, sleep, and minimizing exposure to environmental toxins, all of which play a crucial role in achieving and maintaining health.

Practical tips for daily life, such as maintaining a balanced pH level, reading food labels, and building a support system, are designed to empower readers to make informed, healthful choices. These strategies, along with a detailed herb glossary, FAQs, and resources for further information, provide a comprehensive toolkit for anyone looking to embark on a healing journey based on natural, holistic principles.

By embracing Dr. Sebi's teachings, readers are encouraged to take control of their health, learning to listen to their bodies and make choices that support their well-being. This journey is not just about combating illness, but about thriving in harmony with nature, fostering a life of vitality and wellness.

Encouragement for Your Healing Journey

Your journey towards healing and embracing a life of vitality through Dr. Sebi's teachings is a profound commitment to your well-being. It's a path that unfolds with each step you take, nourishing not just your body, but also your spirit. As you embark on this transformative journey, remember, every change you make, no matter how small, is a powerful act of self-care.

The road to healing is unique for each person and comes with its own set of challenges and triumphs. There may be days when progress seems slow, or the path ahead feels daunting. During these times, it's important to be gentle with yourself, acknowledging the effort it takes to make these life-altering changes. Celebrate every victory, no matter how small, whether it's choosing a healthy meal over processed food, enjoying a moment of peace in nature, or simply taking a deep, cleansing breath.

Remember, you're not alone on this journey. There's a community of like-minded individuals, each with their own stories of healing and transformation, who understand the challenges and rewards of this path. Lean on this community for support, share your experiences, and draw strength from the collective wisdom and encouragement.

Dr. Sebi's principles are more than just guidelines for health; they're a blueprint for living in harmony with nature and your own body. As you integrate these teachings into your life, you'll discover a deeper connection to the world around you and an inner strength you may not have known you possessed. This journey is as much about healing the body as it is about nurturing the soul and fostering a sense of peace and fulfillment.

So, take heart and continue forward with courage and conviction. Your commitment to this healing journey is a testament to your strength and desire for a life of health and vitality. Trust in the process, stay open to learning, and embrace each step with hope and optimism. The path to wellness is a journey of a thousand miles that begins with a single step. Let each step you take be a celebration of life and a step closer to the harmony and health you seek.

Additional Resources and Further Reading

For those inspired to delve deeper into the holistic healing journey and expand their knowledge beyond the scope of this book, a wealth of resources awaits. Exploring additional literature, websites, and community forums can provide further insights into natural health practices, the alkaline diet, and Dr. Sebi's teachings.

Books such as "Alkaline Herbal Medicine" by Aqiyl Aniys offer a comprehensive guide to the use of herbs in the context of an alkaline diet, providing detailed information on herbal remedies that align with Dr. Sebi's principles. "The African Holistic Health" by Dr. Llaila O. Afrika is another invaluable resource, covering a wide range of topics related to holistic African medicine and wellness practices.

Websites like the Dr. Sebi's Cell Food Official Website (drsebiscellfood.com) continue to share Dr. Sebi's legacy, offering articles, products, and testimonials that can inspire and guide individuals on their healing journey. Additionally, platforms such as The National Center for Complementary and Integrative Health (NCCIH) at nccih.nih.gov provide scientifically-based information on various complementary health practices, including herbal supplements and nutritional therapies.

Community forums and social media groups dedicated to alkaline living and natural healing can also be a source of support and information. Platforms like Reddit and Facebook host numerous groups where individuals share their experiences, recipes, and advice related to Dr. Sebi's diet and holistic health in general.

For those interested in the scientific and nutritional aspects of the alkaline diet, academic journals and publications offer research articles and studies that examine the effects of diet on health from a scientific perspective. Websites like PubMed (pubmed.ncbi.nlm.nih.gov) and Google Scholar (scholar.google.com) are excellent starting points for accessing peer-reviewed articles and clinical studies.

By exploring these additional resources and further reading, individuals can deepen their understanding of holistic health, gain new perspectives, and continue to grow in their journey towards wellness. Remember, the path to health is both personal and communal, and there is always more to learn and discover.

Detailed Herb Glossary

Burdock Root: A powerhouse of antioxidants, burdock root is celebrated for its blood purifying properties. It aids in detoxifying the liver, improving skin health, and promoting overall immune system function.

Cinnamon: More than just a spice, cinnamon is revered for its ability to lower blood sugar levels, reduce heart disease risk factors, and its potent antimicrobial properties.

Dandelion: Often considered a weed, dandelion is a valuable herb with roots and leaves that can support liver detoxification, aid digestion, and act as a diuretic to help the body eliminate excess fluid.

Fennel: With a licorice-like taste, fennel is beneficial for digestive health, helping to relieve gas, bloating, and stomach cramps. It's also used to improve eyesight and lower blood pressure.

Ginger: A potent anti-inflammatory and antioxidant, ginger can alleviate nausea, improve digestive health, and may reduce muscle pain and soreness.

Hibiscus: Rich in vitamin C and antioxidants, hibiscus tea can lower blood pressure, support liver health, and help in weight management.

Irish Moss: Also known as Sea Moss, Irish moss is a type of seaweed that's rich in nutrients and antioxidants. It's believed to boost immunity, improve digestion, and hydrate the skin.

Jamaican Dogwood: Used traditionally for its analgesic properties, Jamaican dogwood can help relieve pain, anxiety, and insomnia. It should be used under the guidance of a healthcare professional due to its potent effects.

Kale: While not an herb, kale is included for its exceptional nutrient profile, including vitamins A, C, and K, antioxidants, and minerals. It supports overall health and wellness.

Lavender: Known for its calming and relaxing properties, Lavender can help alleviate stress, improve sleep quality, and support skin health.

Milk Thistle: A liver-supporting herb, Milk Thistle is used to detoxify the liver, promote liver regeneration, and protect against liver damage.

Nettle: Rich in nutrients, Nettle supports urinary tract health, can relieve allergy symptoms, and reduce inflammation.

Oregano: With powerful antimicrobial properties, oregano can help fight infections, improve gut health, and has been used for its antioxidant benefits.

Quinoa: Although a seed, Quinoa is included for its high protein content, complete amino acid profile, and rich mineral content, supporting overall health.

Rosemary: Known for its memory-enhancing properties, Rosemary also supports digestion, improves circulation, and has been used for its anti-inflammatory and antioxidant benefits.

Soursop: Also known as Graviola, Soursop has been used traditionally to fight infections, lower blood pressure, and as a natural remedy for insomnia and stress.

Valerian Root: Used for its sedative properties, Valerian Root can help improve sleep quality, reduce anxiety, and alleviate menstrual cramps.

Wheatgrass: Rich in chlorophyll, vitamins, and minerals, wheatgrass supports detoxification, boosts immunity, and can improve energy levels.

Xanthoparmelia Scabrosa: Often used in traditional medicine to support sexual health, it should be approached with caution and under professional guidance due to limited research.

Yarrow: Known for its ability to stop bleeding and heal wounds, Yarrow also supports digestive health and can reduce symptoms of colds and fevers.

Zinc: Not an herb but included for its critical role in immune function, wound healing, DNA synthesis, and cell division. Zinc is found in various herbs and foods, supporting overall health.

This glossary provides a starting point for understanding the vast world of herbs and their potential benefits. While exploring these natural remedies, remember the importance of consulting with a healthcare professional, especially when managing health conditions or taking other medications, to ensure safety and efficacy in your health journey.

Frequently Asked Questions

Can I start the Dr. Sebi diet if I'm on medication? Absolutely, but it's crucial to consult with your healthcare provider first. The transition to an alkaline diet involves significant changes in your nutritional intake, which could affect how your body responds to medications. Your doctor can guide you on how to safely incorporate these dietary changes alongside your current treatment plan.

How quickly can I expect to see health improvements? Individual experiences vary greatly. Some people report feeling more energetic and experiencing improved digestion within a few days, while for others, noticeable changes may take a few weeks or longer. It's important to listen to your body and give it time to adjust to the new diet.

Is it expensive to follow Dr. Sebi's dietary recommendations? While some of the recommended herbs and supplements can be pricey, the core of the diet—fruits, vegetables, grains, and nuts—can be quite affordable, especially if you choose seasonal and local produce. Planning and preparing meals at home can also help manage costs.

Can I still eat meat on this diet? Dr. Sebi's diet is plant-based and excludes meat, dairy, and processed foods. It focuses on alkaline foods that support the body's pH balance. If eliminating meat entirely is challenging, consider transitioning gradually by reducing meat intake and increasing portions of plant-based foods.

What if I have allergies to some of the recommended foods or herbs? Always prioritize your health and safety. If you're allergic to specific foods or herbs listed in the diet, avoid them. There are plenty of alternative options available that provide similar nutritional benefits. Consulting with a nutritionist or a healthcare provider can help you make suitable adjustments.

Remember, embarking on Dr. Sebi's diet or any significant lifestyle change should be approached with patience and mindfulness. It's about finding balance and what works best for your body.

Resources for Further Information

For those eager to expand their knowledge on natural healing and Dr. Sebi's methodologies, a plethora of resources are available to guide and enrich your journey. Books, websites, and community forums offer a treasure trove of information that can deepen your understanding and application of holistic health principles.

Books like "Mucusless Diet Healing System" by Arnold Ehret and "Back to Eden" by Jethro Kloss provide foundational insights into natural healing and the importance of diet in maintaining health. These works complement Dr. Sebi's teachings and offer historical perspectives on herbal medicine and natural diets.

Websites such as the Dr. Sebi's Cell Food Official Website continue to be a primary source for those following Dr. Sebi's diet, offering not just products, but valuable articles and success stories. Additionally, the National Center for Complementary and Integrative Health provides reliable, research-based information on complementary and alternative medicine, helping readers discern practices supported by scientific evidence.

Community forums and social media platforms are vibrant spaces for sharing experiences and advice. Websites like Reddit have subreddits dedicated to herbal medicine, natural healing, and specific diets like the alkaline diet. Facebook groups and online forums specific to Dr. Sebi's diet offer community support, allowing individuals to share recipes, tips, and personal stories of transformation.

For academic readers, databases like PubMed and Google Scholar are invaluable for accessing peer-reviewed studies on the efficacy of specific herbs, dietary practices, and their impacts on health. These resources can provide a deeper scientific understanding of the principles behind Dr. Sebi's teachings.

Remember, while these resources can offer vast amounts of information, it's essential to approach them with discernment and consider the credibility of the sources. Engaging with a community of like-minded individuals and professionals can also provide support and guidance as you navigate through the wealth of information available on natural healing and holistic health.

Contact Information for Support and Community

For those seeking guidance or wishing to connect with a supportive community as you embark on your journey with Dr. Sebi's healing principles, numerous resources are available. Whether you're looking for professional advice, peer support, or simply wish to share your experiences, reaching out can significantly enhance your journey towards better health.

Professional support can be found through certified holistic health practitioners familiar with Dr. Sebi's methodologies. Many of these professionals offer consultations online, making it easier to access advice regardless of your location. For a list of recommended practitioners, visit the official Dr. Sebi's Cell Food website or contact their customer service for referrals.

Community support plays a crucial role in maintaining motivation and gaining insights from others' experiences. Online forums and social media platforms host vibrant communities dedicated to alkaline living, herbal remedies, and Dr. Sebi's diet. Facebook groups such as "Dr. Sebi's Nutritional Guide" and "Alkaline Plant Based Diet" are excellent places to start. Here, members share recipes, success stories, and tips for navigating challenges.

For those who prefer a more structured support system, several non-profit organizations and wellness centers offer workshops, seminars, and group meetings focused on holistic health and natural healing. These can be valuable opportunities to learn from experienced practitioners and meet like-minded individuals in your area.

Remember, the journey to health is personal but doesn't have to be lonely. Connecting with others can provide the encouragement, knowledge, and support needed to make lasting changes. Whether you're just starting out or have been on this path for a while, there's a community waiting to welcome you.